HAND REFLEXOLOGY & ACUPRESSURE

A Natural Way to Health through
Traditional Chinese Medicine

By Chen Feisong and Gai Guozhong

Better Link Press

This book is edited and designed by the Editorial Committee of *Cultural China* series.

Text by Chen Feisong and Gai Guozhong
Translation by Wu Yanting
Design by Wang Wei

Copy Editor: Susie Gorden
Editorial Assistant: Pei Zhuomin
Editor: Cao Yue
Editorial Director: Zhang Yicong

Senior Consultants: Sun Yong, Wu Ying, Yang Xinci
Managing Director and Publisher: Wang Youbu

ISBN: 978-1-60220-162-0

Address any comments about *Hand Reflexology & Acupressure: A Natural Way to Health through Traditional Chinese Medicine* to:

Better Link Press
99 Park Ave
New York, NY 10016
USA

or

Shanghai Press and Publishing Development Co., Ltd.
F 7 Donghu Road, Shanghai, China (200031)
Email: comments_betterlinkpress@hotmail.com
Printed in China by Shanghai Donnelley Printing Co., Ltd.

1   3   5   7   9   10   8   6   4   2

Contents

Introduction

Human beings are grain-eating creatures, so falling ill at one time or another is inevitable. Therefore, even those of us who are not medical professionals should know something about medicine, nursing the sick, and carrying out emergency treatment. Such knowledge and skills are not confined to physicians. To be sure, we are our own best doctors in terms of taking care of our health.

In recent years, Traditional Chinese Medicine (TCM) has been increasingly acknowledged as an effective way of maintaining good health. According to TCM, the human hand is closely related to the internal organs, meridian channels, and collateral vessels, as well as the neurological system. Hand reflexology and acupressure refer to the practice of using one hand to apply pressure to specific acupoints, pathological reflex points, or sensitive points on the other hand, to help relieve symptoms or heal ailments. Among the various methods of maintaining health, hand reflexology and acupressure do not rely on devices, and incur no toxicity or side effects. They can be used at any time and anywhere. A school of its own, the method is gaining increasing popularity, as it is easy to apply and has immediate effects. It is also quick to learn, economical, and safe.

This book has a simple structure and is easy to use. Chapter One introduces the concept of hand reflexology and acupressure, as well as how it is administered and what to watch out for. Chapter Two expounds on meridians, acupoints and reflex areas with clear illustrations. Chapters Three through Nine deal with 58 common diseases and conditions in the categories of sub-health, circulatory and respiratory systems, neurological and endocrine systems, the digestive system, the urogenital system, gynecology, dermatology, and otorhinolaryngology, and how hand reflexology and acupressure can be applied.

The book has three notable characteristics:

1. It explains complex information in simple language, making it easy to learn. Basic knowledge of hand reflexology and acupressure is offered, and the skills and techniques are also provided to help readers use these methods on their own.

2. It comes with illustrations, detailed instructions, and explanations. A number of illustrations help readers quickly identify the location of acupoints and reflex areas or points in the hand, for ease of practice.

3. The daily care of a variety of diseases and conditions are offered, accompanied by related "hand exercises." Readers can also use these hand exercises independently to help strengthen the dexterity of their fingers for the purpose of maintaining good health.

We hope that this book will give you enough knowledge of hand reflexology and acupressure to become a provider of healthcare for yourself and your family.

Chapter One

Understanding Hand
Reflexology and Acupressure

Published over 2,000 years ago, *Huangdi Neijing* (*The Inner Canon of the Yellow Emperor*) holds that the parts of a human body have a dialectical relationship with the entire bodily system. They are also united: Each part of the body is closely related to the *zang* organs and *fu* organs, meridian channels, and collateral vessels. Hand reflexology and acupressure are alternative medical treatments that take advantage of this theory. The core tenet is that stimulating a related location will stimulate the corresponding organ, facilitating the prevention of diseases and alleviating pain

So what are hand reflexology and acupressure? The concept can be approached in broad and narrow senses.

In a broad sense, hand reflexology and acupressure refer to therapies such as massage, acupuncture, moxibustion, and the application of poultices to the hollow of the palm. Among them, massage therapy is particularly common. It is the easiest to practice and the most economical, and is therefore the most widely used way.

In a narrow sense, hand reflexology and acupressure refer specifically to the application of pressure to related areas and points in the hand for treatment. They include techniques such as jabbing, kneading, pressing, and pushing. By and large, it is a method of applying pressure to pathological reflex points or sensitive spots in the hand that are related to certain organs and tissues inside and outside of the body, in order to heal certain maladies.

There are more than 70 pathological reflex areas and acupoints in the palm and back of a hand where the neurological points gather. Clinical practice shows that accurate application of a specific technique over a period of time will help facilitate positive stimulation of internal organs and help strengthen their function in order to maintain health and prevent the occurrence of certain acute or chronic diseases.

1. Preparation

Hand reflexology and acupressure therapy (hereafter, this term is used specifically in the narrow definition of massaging with fingers) requires no special venue, but enough natural light and little external noise. Before conducting hand reflexology and acupressure, trim your fingernails to about 1 mm long, levelling the flesh tip of the finger, and polish the edges so they are smooth. Long nails tend to scratch the skin, but if they are too short, they may not produce the required effect.

As acupoints in the hand occupy tiny spaces, the use of small tools (such as sticks, cotton swabs, ballpoint pens, and other pens) is recommended for easy administration. Please do not use sharp objects.

Tools you need:

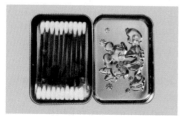

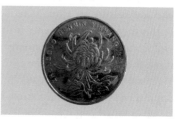

Cotton swabs: In order to execute pressure more accurately to an acupoint on the hand, you may use a match stick or a cotton swab. Make sure that the stick does not have a sharp end so that it doesn't hurt the skin. You may also use the shaft of a pen.

Coin: For use in the hand exercises in this book. While doing hand exercises, you may also use other objects such as a toothbrush, a wristwatch, or a small ball.

2. Benefits

- **Widely applicable:** It can relieve symptoms of various diseases and conditions, and can promote good health. Many common diseases and conditions in clinical departments (such as internal medicine, orthopedics, gynecology, dermatology, and otolaryngology) can be prevented or alleviated by applying hand reflexology and acupressure therapy.
- **Safe and reliable:** Free of trauma and side effects, no pollution, no medical dependency, and no harm done to the *fu* organs and *zang* organs.
- **Easy to learn and administer:** No complicated medical devices are needed. Your hand alone is the tool of administration, supplemented by simple everyday objects. The techniques are easy to master, and you can do them anywhere and anytime. It is perfect for domestic health care and the prevention of diseases.
- **Effective:** Applicable to a variety of conditions, and usually has surprisingly positive results as long as it is administered properly. In addition, hand reflexology and acupressure therapy can be tools for

the maintenance and promotion of heath. As long as you keep doing it, you will be amazed at how much you will be benefited.

3. Points of Attention

- Apply pressure appropriately. Press each acupoint or reflex area for 3 to 5 minutes. Each session should last between 15 and 30 minutes. For acute diseases and conditions, administer once or twice daily and stop once healed. For chronic diseases and conditions, administer once daily or every other day, and 5 to 10 times as a course of treatment. Follow the sequential numbers to massage your hands for each disease.

- Acupoints are symmetrically distributed in both hands. When you have finished pressing the acupoints on one hand, repeat on the other hand.

- Do not apply hand reflexology or acupressure on a full stomach, or when hungry or extremely fatigued. Take a 15-minute rest before hand reflexology and acupressure therapy. Take a 30-minute rest after high-impact exercise. Do not perform hand reflexology or acupressure therapy until one hour after a bath.

- For the elderly, whose knuckles tend to be stiff and whose bones become porous and brittle, massages should be soft and gentle. Avoid applying too strong a force.

- Do not perform hand reflexology or acupressure if there is any inflection or festering growth in the hand. Be cautious with sensitive skin.

- Some people may feel slight pain, soreness, and swelling after the first treatment. This is due to over-exertion of force, so force should to be reduced in the next session.

- Relax and breathe with ease during the therapy session. Do not hold your breath.

- Acupoints in the hand usually occupy tiny spaces, so you may want to use small objects such as match stick, cotton swab, ball-pointed pen, or pen to help administer pressure to these points. Do not use pointed objects for this purpose.

- Keep warm in winter, and avoid exposing your hands to low temperatures in case of blisters. In summer when the weather is humid, use an electric fan to reduce the heat, but avoid blowing directly at the person. Hand reflexology and acupressure therapy are best conducted in a ventilated place.

- To those with more serious diseases and conditions, hand reflexology and acupressure therapy work best in combination with regular medical treatment. Alternatively, you can use hand reflexology and acupressure as a supplement to regular medical treatment in order to expedite recovery.

• The hand exercises in this book are complementary to hand reflexology and acupressure. After finishing with one hand, do the same with the other.

4. Techniques for Administration

There are ten basic hand reflexology and acupressure techniques, including pressing, kneading, jabbing, twisting, pinching, pushing, rubbing in straight lines, and rubbing in circular motion. Each technique is applicable to certain points, and the points you should pay attention to are provided, to assist you with the therapy. The following are the eight most commonly used techniques.

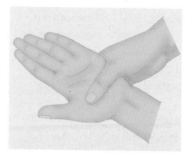

Pressing

Definition: Use the tip of the thumb or the tip of the finger to press. The force is administered from the top down, to the acupoint, reflex area, and reaction point.

Applicable to: Flatter zones such as the thenar eminence (*da yuji*) and hypothenar eminence (*xiao yuji*). This method is often combined with kneading to prevent or alleviate some chronic diseases and chronic pain.

Attention: Wherever you apply force, make sure that your fingers are closely pressed to the surface of the hand and move in a limited range. The force applied should be incremental, slow and steady. Avoid abrupt bursts of force, evening out the frequency and the force of pressure.

Kneading

Definition: Put the tip of the finger on the point or area of the hand, relax your wrist; using your elbow as a point of support, vacillate the forearm to move the wrist and the metacarpus to knead softly and gently in a circular motion, so the pressure will be transmitted

to designated places through
the fingers. The middle finger
and the thumb are used most
commonly for kneading.

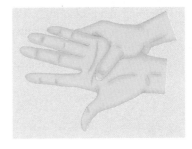

Applicable to: Toning the
body's constitution. It is better
to apply the force to more
superficial acupoints or open
acupoints. Kneading is usually
used to alleviate symptoms of chronic diseases, deficiency syndromes,
and consumptive diseases.

Attention: The force should be applied gently. The administration
is coordinated and rhythmic. Better to do it for a sustained period of
time, about one half time longer than the regular treatment.

Jabbing

Definition: Use the tip of the
thumb, the tip of the middle
finger, the tip of the ulnar
side of the little finger, the
tip of the ring finger, and the
interphalangeal joint to jab the
acupoints in the hand.

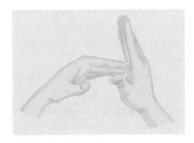

Applicable to: Areas and
points between the bones. Often used for treatment of acute diseases
and pain.

Attention: Jabbing touches only tiny spots of the hand, but the
pressure is powerful and therefore has a strong impact. Make sure your
administration is straight to the point, and do not slip.

Twisting

Definition: Use the tips of your
thumb and index finger to pinch
a specific location and then twist
it. This method helps facilitate
blood circulation, clear the
channels, and alleviate pain.

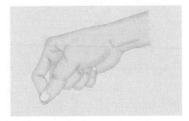

Applicable to: All the joints
of your hands. Often used for chronic diseases and local discomfort, or

maintaining and promoting good health.

Attention: Adequate frequency and degrees of force are stressed. Adjust the frequency and force of pressure depending on how the patient feels during a hand reflexology or acupressure session.

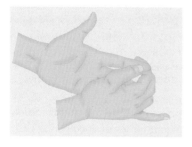

Pinching

Definition: Use the tip of the fingernail to apply strong force to points or areas in the hand. Usually, the tip of the thumb and the radius side of its nail edge are used to apply force, or the thumb works with the tips of all the other fingernail tips to pinch the points or areas and apply force to the place they pinch.

Applicable to: Usually where the metacarpus knuckles connect the fingers, and between the metacarpus of the palm. Often used for alleviating pain, the onset of manic syndrome, acute diseases, and neurasthenia.

Attention: Pinching is a method that produces a strong impact. Therefore, apply force incrementally and stop as soon as there is an intense reaction. Do not slip when administering force, or you may scrape the skin. To avoid scraping the skin, cover it with a piece of thin cloth when intense pinching is to be administered.

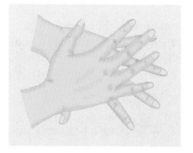

Pushing

Definition: Use the palm and fingers, a single finger, multiple fingers and the heel of the palm, the thenar eminence, or the hypothenar eminence to apply force to specific acupoints and reflex points. Push in one direction in a straight line.

Applicable to: Push longitudinally in the hand. Rubbing in straight lines is usually added after pushing has been administered for a period of time. Pushing is often used to treat chronic diseases, alleviate pain and soreness caused by strain or wear and tear, conditions of cold deficiency, and maintaining good health.

Attention: When pushing, keep the fingers and the palm flat, securely press them to the skin, and apply adequate force. Do it slowly and evenly to maintain good control of the force. Pushing is usually administered in the orientation of the bones of the hand.

Rubbing (in straight lines)

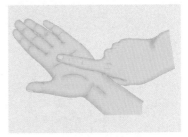

Definition: Use a single finger, the palm, the thenar eminence and hypothenar eminence, or the heel of the palm to press a specific location on the hand, and move in a straight line back and forth in quick motion.

Applicable to: Along the bone orientation of the palm and fingers, particularly the center of the palm. This is beneficial for conditions such as chronic diseases, cold deficient syndrome, and mental illnesses. It is also recommended for promoting physical fitness.

Attention: The wrist joint stretches out naturally when relaxed. Your forearm and hand are on the same level, with the fingertips pressing down slightly. The administration of force is light but not superficial, with a quick rhythm.

Rubbing (in circular motion)

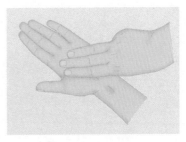

Definition: Press the palm or the tips of the index finger, middle finger, and ring finger to a specific location on the hand, and move your wrist joint as well as your forearm at the point or area in your hand to rub in circular motion, clockwise or counter-clockwise.

Applicable to: More open locations on the hand. Often used to alleviate age-related diseases, chronic diseases, deficient syndrome, and cold syndrome.

Attention: Rapid rhythm is required, but the movement should be gentle and the speed even. Avoid irregular and heavy-handed rubbing, which will compromise the result.

Chapter Two

Acupoints and
Reflex Points and Areas
in the Hand

B efore explaining hand reflexology or acupressure, this chapter aims to provide readers with a brief introduction to the concepts of the meridian system and the holographic reflex areas in Traditional Chinese Medicine. The two concepts, though belonging to different theoretical systems, are complementary to each other, and play a crucial role in hand reflexology and acupressure, according to TCM.

1. Meridians and Acupoints

As the basis of TCM theory, the meridian system can actually be felt in real life. However, no research has so far found any convincing evidence of its physical form. To put it simply, the meridian system is like a traffic network spreading across the human body, consisting of channels designed exclusively to supply *qi* (vital energy) and blood to every part of the body. Among them, the principal channels are called *jing* (meridians), whereas the branching vessels connecting the principal channels and connected with one another are called *luo* (collateral). Serving the five visceral organs (*wuzang*) and six bowel organs (*liufu*), they crisscross the human body, connecting the surface and the depth as well as the top and the bottom as an organic whole. Through the circulation of *qi* and blood, they provide nutrition to sustain the organic livelihood of the human body.

There are fourteen meridians in the human body. They are:
- Taiyin Lung Meridian of the Hand (LU);
- Yangming Large Intestine Meridian of the Hand (LI);
- Yangming Stomach Meridian of the Foot (ST);
- Taiyin Spleen Meridian of the Foot (SP);
- Shaoyin Heart Meridian of the Hand (HT);
- Taiyang Small Intestine Meridian of the Hand (SI);
- Taiyang Bladder Meridian of the Foot (BL);
- Shaoyin Kidney Meridian of the Foot (KI);
- Jueyin Pericardium Meridian of the Hand (PC);
- Shaoyang Sanjiao Meridian of the Hand (TE);
- Shaoyang Gallbladder Meridian of the Foot (GB);
- Jueyin Liver Meridian of the Foot (LR);
- Conception Vessel (CV);
- Governing Vessel (GV).

The hand is traversed by a large number of meridians. The fingers, as the human body's upper extremities, are one of the places where blood flow starts to go back into the body. Moreover, meridians pertaining to such organs as the heart, lung, large intestine, the triple energizer (*sanjiao*) and pericardium (fig. 1) all go through the fingers and have some points there. Therefore, fingers are believed to correspond to the internal organs: The thumb reflects the functions of the lung and the spleen; the index finger the stomach and the intestines; the middle finger the cardiovascular functions; the ring finger the liver and the gallbladder; and the little finger the uterus, testicles, and kidneys.

Massaging related fingers will help to alleviate symptoms of some diseases:

- Taiyin Lung Meridian of the Hand (thumb): For pneumonia, shortness of breath, coughing, tightness of chest, and nosebleeds.
- Yangming Large Intestine Meridian of the Hand (index finger): For abdominal pain, diarrhea, enteritis, toothache, rhinitis, headaches, and anxiety.
- Jueyin Pericardium Meridian of the Hand (middle finger): For chest pain, irritability, tightness of chest, dizziness, and diabetes.
- Shaoyang Sanjiao Meridian of the Hand (SJ) (ring finger): For migraine, vertigo, and indigestion.
- Shaoyin Heart Meridian of the Hand (HT) (little finger): For palpitations, chest pain, and manic syndrome.

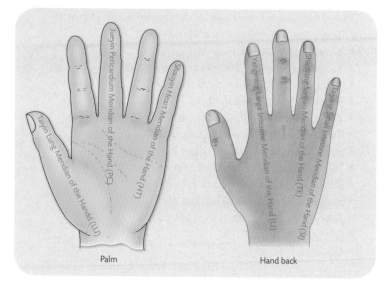

Fig. 1 Organs such as the heart, lungs, large intestine, the triple energizer (*sanjiao*), pericardium, and small intestine all have meridians that pass through the fingers.

- Taiyang Small Intestine Meridian of the Hand (SI) (little finger): For breast pain, ENT diseases, ophthalmological and dental issues, and insufficient breast milk secretion.

Located along the pathways of the meridian and collateral, acupoints are usually places where nerve endings concentrate, or locations where thicker nerve fibers travel. When you feel discomfort or pain, it is the acupoints that send out such signals. The acupoints situated along the pathways of the fourteen principal meridians are called "meridian points." In addition, there are acupoints in certain fixed location that have special effects for treatment. Those are called "extra-ordinary points." These acupoints are not isolated on the surface of your skin, but are closely related to organs and tissues deep in your body.

Therefore, in a sense, acupoints reflect problems in your body, and are working points for treating those problems (figs. 2–3):

- **Shangyang** (LI 1): For toothache, and painful or swollen throat.
- **Erjian** (LI 2): For cranial nerve injuries, eczema, allergic rhinitis, acute conjunctivitis (or pink eye), and constipation.
- **Hegu** (LI 4): For chronic gastritis, menstrual cramps, irregular periods, urticaria, and cataract.
- **Yangxi** (LI 5): For headaches, hearing loss, tinnitus, headache due to reversed upward flow of *qi*, tightness in the chest and shortness of breath, painful and swollen red eyes, ENT-related diseases, ophthalmological and dental problems, stroke, hemiplegia, and problems with wrist joints and surrounding soft tissues.
- **Daling** (PC 7): For anemia, hypotension, irritability, and headache.
- **Laogong** (PC 8): For jaundice, chest pain, tightness in the chest, insomnia, nausea, vomiting, irritability, and restlessness.
- **Zhongchong** (PC 9): For loss of consciousness, sun stroke, faintness, nocturnal fretfulness in infants, and stiffness, swelling and pain in the tongue.
- **Guanchong** (TE 1): For indigestion in infants.
- **Zhongzhu** (TE 3): For nosebleeds, gingivitis, facial paralysis, trigeminal neuralgia, abdominal sounds, and toothache.
- **Yangchi** (TE 4): For loss of hearing and unquenchable thirst.
- **Shenmen** (HT 7): For irritability, fretfulness, insomnia, anemia, and hypotension.
- **Shaochong** (HT 9): For palpitations, chest pain, manic syndrome, and coma.

- **Shaoze** (SI 1): For breast pain, ENT diseases, ophthalmological and dental problems, and insufficient breast milk secretion.
- **Qian'gu** (SI 2): For headache, pain in the eye and ear, painful and swollen throat, insufficient breast milk secretion, and heat pathogen diseases.
- **Houxi** (SI 3): For loss of hearing, manic syndrome, and malaria.
- **Wan'gu** (SI 4): For diabetes and cholecystitis.
- **Yanggu** (SI 5): For tinnitus, stomatitis, parotitis (mumps), and epilepsy.
- **Yanglao** (SI 6): For myopia, stiff neck, mental and neurological disorders, and sequelae of cerebrovascular disease.

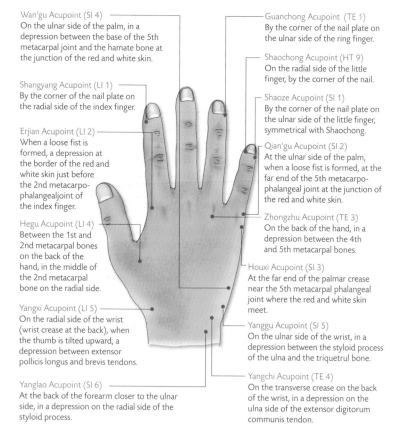

Wan'gu Acupoint (SI 4)
On the ulnar side of the palm, in a depression between the base of the 5th metacarpal joint and the hamate bone at the junction of the red and white skin.

Shangyang Acupoint (LI 1)
By the corner of the nail plate on the radial side of the index finger.

Erjian Acupoint (LI 2)
When a loose fist is formed, a depression at the border of the red and white skin just before the 2nd metacarpo-phalangealjoint of the index finger.

Hegu Acupoint (LI 4)
Between the 1st and 2nd metacarpal bones on the back of the hand, in the middle of the 2nd metacarpal bone on the radial side.

Yangxi Acupoint (LI 5)
On the radial side of the wrist (wrist crease at the back), when the thumb is tilted upward, a depression between extensor pollicis longus and brevis tendons.

Yanglao Acupoint (SI 6)
At the back of the forearm closer to the ulnar side, in a depression on the radial side of the styloid process.

Guanchong Acupoint (TE 1)
By the corner of the nail plate on the ulnar side of the ring finger.

Shaochong Acupoint (HT 9)
On the radial side of the little finger, by the corner of the nail.

Shaoze Acupoint (SI 1)
By the corner of the nail plate on the ulnar side of the little finger, symmetrical with Shaochong.

Qian'gu Acupoint (SI 2)
At the ulnar side of the palm, when a loose fist is formed, at the far end of the 5th metacarpo-phalangeal joint at the junction of the red and white skin.

Zhongzhu Acupoint (TE 3)
On the back of the hand, in a depression between the 4th and 5th metacarpal bones.

Houxi Acupoint (SI 3)
At the far end of the palmar crease near the 5th metacarpal phalangeal joint where the red and white skin meet.

Yanggu Acupoint (SI 5)
On the ulnar side of the wrist, in a depression between the styloid process of the ulna and the triquetrul bone.

Yangchi Acupoint (TE 4)
On the transverse crease on the back of the wrist, in a depression on the ulna side of the extensor digitorum communis tendon.

Fig. 2 Acupoints on the back of the hand.

- **Lieque** (LU 7): For coughing, shortness of breath, painful and swollen throat, headaches, toothache, and Bell's palsy.
- **Yuji** (LU 10): For chronic bronchitis and tonsillitis.
- **Taiyuan** (LU 9): For colds, shortness of breath, chest pain, painful and swollen throat, and allergic rhinitis.
- **Shaoshang** (LU 11): For pharyngitis, acute pneumonia, high fever, and difficulty breathing.

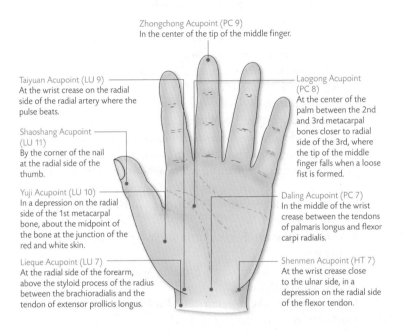

Zhongchong Acupoint (PC 9)
In the center of the tip of the middle finger.

Taiyuan Acupoint (LU 9)
At the wrist crease on the radial side of the radial artery where the pulse beats.

Shaoshang Acupoint (LU 11)
By the corner of the nail at the radial side of the thumb.

Yuji Acupoint (LU 10)
In a depression on the radial side of the 1st metacarpal bone, about the midpoint of the bone at the junction of the red and white skin.

Lieque Acupoint (LU 7)
At the radial side of the forearm, above the styloid process of the radius between the brachioradialis and the tendon of extensor prollicis longus.

Laogong Acupoint (PC 8)
At the center of the palm between the 2nd and 3rd metacarpal bones closer to radial side of the 3rd, where the tip of the middle finger falls when a loose fist is formed.

Daling Acupoint (PC 7)
In the middle of the wrist crease between the tendons of palmaris longus and flexor carpi radialis.

Shenmen Acupoint (HT 7)
At the wrist crease close to the ulnar side, in a depression on the radial side of the flexor tendon.

Fig. 3 Acupoints in the palm of the hand.

2. Reflex Points and Areas

Hologram theory in TCM draws on hologram science, bio-hologram theory, and traditional Chinese theories. It combines both Western and Chinese medical sciences, and offers a window into the developments of the human body in a dynamic and straightforward manner.

Hologram theory holds that a human body is an organic whole. Any changes in physiological functions, and pathological changes in a local organ will have an impact on the overall function and pathological state of the human body. An imbalance of overall function will inevitably affect all of the organs. Therefore, when treating a disease in a local organ, we should make an effort to tune the overall balance of the body. When treating systemic diseases, we should try to stimulate local organs as well. There are many holographic reflex areas and points in the hand that pertain to the internal organs and tissues of the human body. These reflex areas play a unique and independent role in addition to the meridian points and extra-ordinary points.

According to hologram theory, stimulating the reflex points and areas in the hand can prevent or heal some diseases. The movements provided by the two hands will transmit positive stimulation to the organs, balance the *yin* and *yang*, and promote the circulation of *qi* and blood, which in turn will boost physical fitness.

The following are some examples of reflex areas in the hand (fig. 4), elucidating the positive effects each reflex area has on specific diseases.

- (Light blue area) Chest & respiratory organs: For cold, asthma, coughing, painful and swollen throat, congested nose.
- (Red area) Stomach, spleen & large intestine: For loss of appetite, acne, obesity, acute and chronic enteritis.
- (Dark pink area) Reproduction: For abnormal menstruation, menopause syndrome, spermatorrhea, sexual dysfunction.
- (Green area) Ear & throat: For laryngeal foreign bodies, otitis media, vertigo.
- (Yellow area) Palm: For neurasthenia, insomnia, autonomic nerve disorders.
- (Light pink area) Essence & heart: For heart disease, insomnia, difficulty breathing.
- (Dark green area) Gastrointestine: For loss of appetite, indigestion, diarrhea.
- (Dark blue area)Foot&leg:For lower back pain, leg pain, foot pain.
- (Purple area) Palm center: For aversion to cold, anemia, carsickness, loss of appetite.
- (Orange area) Liver & gallbladder: For diseases of the liver and the gallbladder, toothache, headache, eye fatigue, urticaria.

The hand's reflex points and areas all play roles in alleviating the symptoms of specific diseases. For example, massaging the heart point will relieve symptoms of headache and anxiety; massaging the kidney point will alleviate symptoms of toothache, and diseases of the kidney and the bladder; massaging the cough & asthma point will help ease asthma and coughing.

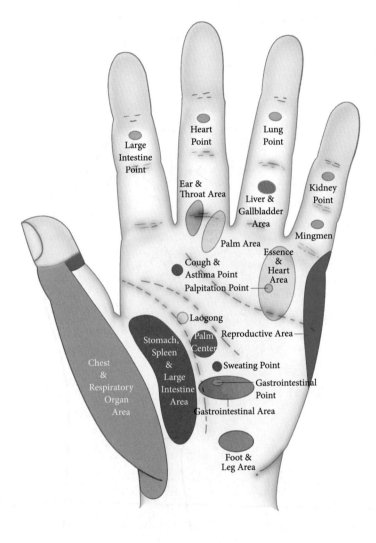

Fig. 4 Reflex points and areas in the palm.

The reflex points and areas located on the side and the back of the hand (figs. 5–6) all have an impact on specific organs and diseases, which are explained later in the book. In the subsequent chapters, we will explain how to alleviate the symptoms of diseases by massaging the related points and areas as suggested by acupoints in TCM and the theory of holographic reflection.

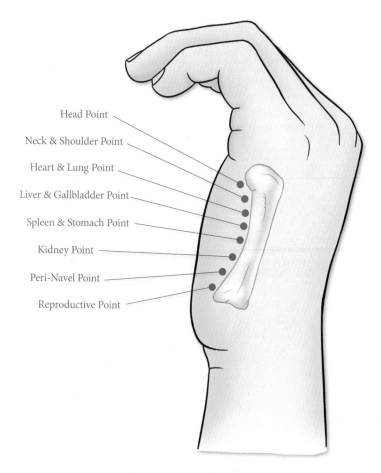

Head Point
Neck & Shoulder Point
Heart & Lung Point
Liver & Gallbladder Point
Spleen & Stomach Point
Kidney Point
Peri-Navel Point
Reproductive Point

Fig. 5 Reflex points of the fifth metacarpus.

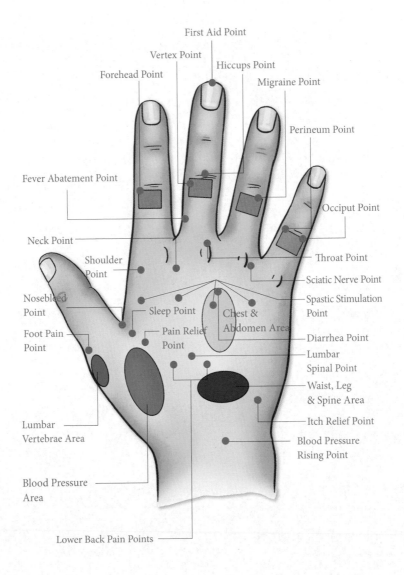

Fig. 6 Reflex points and areas on the back of the hand.

Chapter Three

Sub-Health Conditions

Suboptimal health (or sub-health) status refers to an intermediate state between health and disease. It is characterized by conditions such as lower back pain, insomnia, and constipation. Although they are not exactly diseases, they affect the quality of life, and result in emotional stress at work. They will eventually drain a person's vitality. Hand reflexology and acupressure are accessible and effective means of improving these conditions, conducted either in the office or at home.

1. Lower Back Pain

Lower back pain refers to the pain one feels on one or both sides of the lower back, or pain involving the back and the spine. It can also trigger pain in the lower abdomen, or a painful sensation involving the hipbones and legs.

There is a variety of reasons for lower back pain. Most often, it is caused by kidney deficiency, herniated lumbar disc or swollen disc, degenerated lumbar muscles, lumbar hyperplasia, lumbar spinal stenosis, and diseases of the reproductive organs. Women suffering from diseases such as rheumatism and rheumatoid arthritis are susceptible to lower back pain triggered by vertebral hyperosteogeny resulting from invasion of wind, dampness, and cold during menstrual periods, childbirth, and post-partum periods. It may also be triggered by fatigue during pregnancy and the puerperal period.

Manifestations and Symptoms

In the elderly, lower back pain caused by degenerative problems in the joints can have the following manifestations: Lower back pain and stiffness, which may worsen after some rest, during the night, or when getting up in the morning, but may subside after some activities; excessive activity or heavy fatigue will worsen lower back pain; when the weather is cold or damp, the pain may be aggravated.

Signs of lower back pain caused by strain or sprain are as follows: The pain becomes so severe that the sufferer is afraid of coughing and deep breathing; some may not even be able to stand up. In this case, the point of pain is often identifiable when pressed.

Lower back pain caused by strain on the soft tissues has the following signs: Dull pain, distending pain, and soreness; the points of pain have fixed locations.

Lower back pain in pregnancy: During pregnancy, as the fetus grows, the mother may suffer from lower back pain because of softened ligaments in the lumbosacral region; also, the increasing weight of the fetus puts a lot of pressure on the uterus, so the center of the body tends to tip forward and the lower back protrudes forward. A lack of rest can make a pregnant woman susceptible to lower back pain.

Hand Reflexology and Acupressure

❶ Lumbar Spinal Point
Jab 20 times

❸ Sciatic Nerve Point
Jab 20 times

❷ Lower Back Pain Points
Jab 20 times

❹ Taiyuan Acupoint (LU 9)
Rub in circular motion 20 times

Hand Exercises

① ② ③

1. Open your palm; abruptly bring the middle finger down to the thumb while keeping the index finger, ring finger, and little finger straight.

2. Use your right thumb and index finger to pinch the skin at the root of the left index finger along its metacarpal bone line extension.

3. With the palm facing inward, bring the tip of the middle finger down to press the root of the middle finger. Bend the remaining four fingers inward to form a fist, and bend the thumb to hold the ring finger so the middle finger does not close in too much, forming a fist with the knuckle of the middle finger sticking out.

Other Methods

Particularly susceptible to lower back pain are those who work long hours sitting down, drive or bend over for extended periods, maintain a fixed position in their waist at work, and women with extremely thin waists. These people should take preventive measures, such as keeping their backs in the right position, avoiding excessive fatigue, preventing external trauma to the back, avoiding the invasion of cold in this area, and exercising the back muscles to make them stronger.

Pregnant women can use a belly belt or a belt designed exclusively to support their backs. Avoid standing up abruptly. When standing up, hold on to a table or a chair for support to prevent an excessive burden on the back. These measures will effectively decrease the chances of lower back pain.

2. Headache

A common clinical symptom, headache is a subjective sensation brought about by various pain factors. It often happens in the upper half of the head, above the brows, the upper part of the helix, and the external occipital protuberance. Headache involves a number of systems, and is often associated with neurological diseases.

The causes of headache vary, but they are generally divided into primary headache and secondary headache. Primary headache is not a symptom of an underlying disease, and often manifests as a tension-type headache or migraine. Secondary headache is usually associated with pathological changes in the head and body.

Manifestations and Symptoms

Headaches vary greatly in severity, and last for different periods of time.

They come in a variety of forms. Most commonly they are dull, distending, electrifying, splitting, tearing, and pricking. They are sometimes accompanied by a pulsing of the blood vessels and compression of the head, as well as nausea, vomiting, and dizziness.

Extreme headaches may result in the loss of ability for life and work.

Hand Reflexology and Acupressure

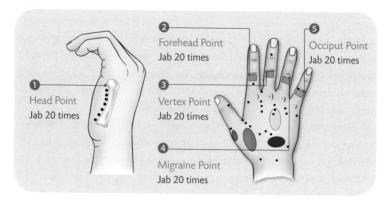

① Head Point
Jab 20 times

② Forehead Point
Jab 20 times

③ Vertex Point
Jab 20 times

④ Migraine Point
Jab 20 times

⑤ Occiput Point
Jab 20 times

Hand Exercises

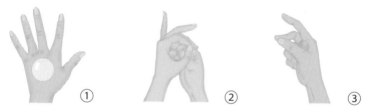

① ② ③

1. Place a ball on the back of your hand and roll it back and forth, left and right.

2. Gather the five digits of your right hand together and wrap them in the palm of your left hand. Squeeze and release them repeatedly.

3. Bend the five digits of your right hand to form a hollow fist; align the thumb with the middle finger and these fingertips jab against each other.

Other Methods

Those who suffer from headaches can also alleviate them with a change of lifestyle:

1. Choose a quiet environment and a room with gentle lighting.

2. Drink tea that is conducive to relieving headache. e.g., tea made with the white bulb of a scallion and Sichuan lovage rhizome, and tea made with chrysanthemum flowers and angelica dahurica.

To make tea with the white bulb of a scallion and Sichuan lovage rhizome: Take two lengths of white scallion, 10 g Sichuan lovage, and

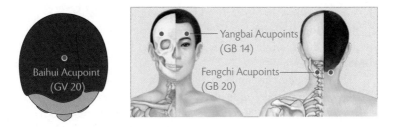

10 g tea leaves. Put them in a cup, pour in boiling water and let it rest, then remove the solids and drink the tea while it is warm. Drink once daily. This tea helps to dispel wind from body and relieve pain.

To make tea with chrysanthemum flowers and angelica dahurica: Take 9 g chrysanthemum flowers and 9 g angelica dohurica; grind them to powder; pour in boiling water, stir, and drink. This tea helps to dispel wind and sooth the liver, and also relieves involuntary muscle spasm and pain.

3. Treatment by massage. Work on Yangbai acupoints (GB 14) if the headache occurs in the forehead; on Baihui acupoint (GV 20) if the headache occurs on the sides; on Fengchi acupoints (GB 20) if the headache happens on the vertex.

3. Insomnia

Insomnia is defined as trouble falling asleep or trouble remaining asleep. It is often accompanied by a lack of energy in the daytime, slow responses, physical weakness, and fatigue. When severe, it affects the everyday life of the person affected.

It can be caused by physical discomforts or unhealthy habits such as drinking strong tea and coffee before bed and smoking. Negative factors in life, such as struggling with conflicting thoughts, stress from work, difficulties in studies, loss of hope, and the departure of loved ones, or even positive factors such as jubilation from success can also cause insomnia. This is referred to as "insomnia due to mental stress." Excessive excitement or worries due to particular events will cause "opportunistic insomnia," resulting in an inadequate amount of sleep.

Manifestations and Symptoms
Difficulty falling asleep or remaining asleep; waking up easily during

the night; waking up too early and not being able to fall asleep again; waking up feeling unrefreshed and fatigued; waking up frequently due to nightmares or the feeling of having nightmares throughout the night.

The duration of insomnia varies. For some, it is over within a few days, but for others, difficulty sleeping may persist and normal sleep may never return. Severe insomnia can worsen or trigger other conditions such as palpitations, chest pain due to blockage in the blood vessels leading to your heart, dizziness, headaches, and stroke.

Hand Reflexology and Acupressure

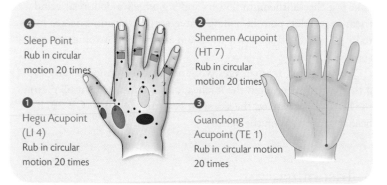

4 Sleep Point
Rub in circular motion 20 times

2 Shenmen Acupoint (HT 7)
Rub in circular motion 20 times

1 Hegu Acupoint (LI 4)
Rub in circular motion 20 times

3 Guanchong Acupoint (TE 1)
Rub in circular motion 20 times

Hand Exercises

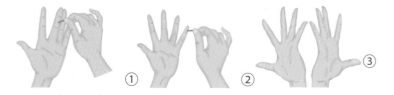

1. Use a stick to jab the palm side of the middle finger evenly, with the stick leaning towards the fingertip.

2. Use a stick to jab the little finger evenly, starting from the tip along the metacarpal bone.

3. Spread the fingers out, and turn the backs of the hands against each other.

Other Methods

1. Do not overeat at dinner. Avoid stimulating drinks such as tea and coffee before sleep. Maintain a diet that is light and rich in protein and vitamins.

2. Create a quiet and comfortable environment that is conducive to good sleep. Prepare a bed of adequate firmness for you to sleep on, and a pillow of adequate height for your neck.

3. Have a fixed bedtime and make it into a routine. Always do the same thing before going to bed: e.g., take a hot bath, and then read for ten minutes before trying to fall asleep. Soon your brain will be tuned to sleep. These activities will help to induce the sleepiness you need.

4. If you cannot fall asleep within 30 minutes, get up and go to another room and sit quietly for 20 minutes before going back to your room to sleep. If you still cannot fall asleep, do the same a few more times until you fall asleep.

4. Vertigo

Vertigo refers to dizziness, blurred vision, or blackout, when you feel that your surroundings are spinning or moving, and you cannot stand still.

Faintness and a spinning sensation are often symptoms of neural dysfunction in the brain. If it happens only once in a while, it could be the result of staying up late at night, excessive use of the brain, or poor ventilation in the room causing inadequate oxygen intake. If it happens constantly, it may be associated with conditions such as anemia, hypoglycemia, orthostatic hypotension, high blood pressure, arteriosclerosis, reduced intracranial pressure, neurasthenia, cerebral thrombosis, rhinitis, and side effects of medication. Many diseases will share symptoms with vertigo. It is important that you seek proper medical advice.

Manifestations and Symptoms

Vertigo falls into the following categories:

Spinning: A false sense that the sky and the ground are spinning.

Syncope: Often occurs when you yank your head backward suddenly, or stand up suddenly from a sitting position.

Floating: Feeling as if you are standing on a pile of cotton.

Shaking: Feeling like an earthquake, moving up and down.

Hand Reflexology and Acupressure

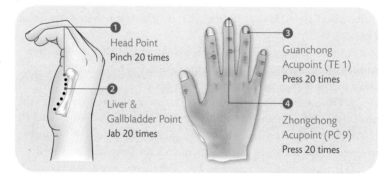

1 Head Point
Pinch 20 times

2 Liver &
Gallbladder Point
Jab 20 times

3 Guanchong
Acupoint (TE 1)
Press 20 times

4 Zhongchong
Acupoint (PC 9)
Press 20 times

Hand Exercises

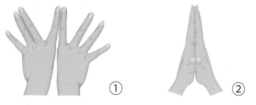

① ②

1. With your palms down, withdraw the thumbs and keep the two hands attached side by side. Abruptly spread out the remaining four fingers. The move should be explosive.

2. Put your palms upright, facing each other; stretch the thumbs towards you; the two palms push against each other with force, and the fingertips swing from left to right six times while the palms are in confrontation.

Other Methods

1. At the onset of vertigo, the patient should lie down, relax, and be free of all emotional tensions.

2. The patient is advised to eat light, fresh, and nutritious food, and refrain from stimulating drinks such as alcohol and coffee. Eat more fruit that is rich in Vitamin C, such as lemons, grapes, and kiwi fruits; eat more eggs, lean meat, and green vegetables. Avoid spicy and fatty food such as fatty meat, fried food, alcohol, and hot chili pepper.

3. Pay attention to mental health, as emotional stress and anger can trigger vertigo. The patient should develop a broad mind, be happy and optimistic, and maintain emotional stability.

4. Avoid excessive fatigue or inadequate sleep.

5. Shock ....

Shock can be caused by such events as external trauma, loss of blood, burns, extreme emotional stimulants, and fear. If left untreated, the patient can suffer from loss of consciousness or a sudden drop in body temperature. Worse still, the patient may die.

Manifestations and Symptoms
Shock is an emergency cardiac and circulatory malfunction. Common clinical manifestations include low blood pressure, weak pulse, cold and clammy limps, grey-bluish skin, and a state of delirium.

Hand Reflexology and Acupressure

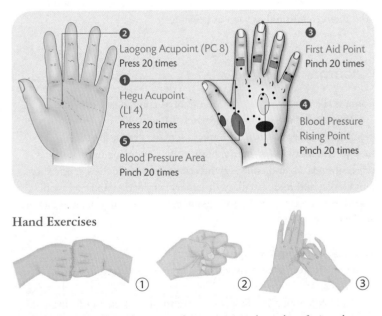

② Laogong Acupoint (PC 8)
Press 20 times

③ First Aid Point
Pinch 20 times

① Hegu Acupoint
(LI 4)
Press 20 times

④ Blood Pressure
Rising Point
Pinch 20 times

⑤ Blood Pressure Area
Pinch 20 times

Hand Exercises

① ② ③

1. Close your hands to form two fists; position the palms facing down, and interlock the knuckles so they press against the depressions of the other hand, and press hard against each other.

2. With the palm facing inward, fold the middle finger so the fingertip touches its root; then bring the remaining four fingers inward to form a fist, and bend the thumb to stop the middle finger closing in too much, thus forming a fist with the middle finger's

knuckle sticking out.

3. With the right thumb and index finger, pinch and pull the skin on the back of the left index finger along its metacarpal bone until you reach the wrist crease.

Other Methods

1. When you see someone in shock, first calm them down and offer some emotional comfort.

2. If the patient is feeling cold, move them to a warmer place and cover them with a quilt. Make them lie down to rest with their feet elevated.

3. If the person feels nauseous, push their head to the side to stop them from choking on their own vomit. If they feels thirsty, give them some warm water or sugary drink. If they are in a severe condition, take them to hospital as soon as possible.

6. Coma

Coma is the most severe stage of impaired consciousness.

It occurs in the following diseases: Intracranial infections such as meningitis, encephalitis, and brain abscesses; cranial brain disorders such as traumatic brain injury, brain tumor, parasitic brain diseases, cerebral malaria, and epilepsy; infectious diseases such as septic shock, septicemia, and toxic bacillary dysentery; endocrine and metabolic disorders such as thyroid disorders, hepatic coma, uremia, and diabetic ketoacidosis.

Manifestations and Symptoms

Different degrees of unconsciousness in a coma have different symptoms:

Mild coma: Some responses to intense stimulation inducing pain; basic physiological responses (swallowing, coughing, corneal reflection, reaction of the pupil to light) and vital signs of life, but may be accompanied by delirium and restlessness.

Moderate coma: No response to pain stimulation but basic physiological responses exist, and there are vital signs of life.

Severe coma: Except for vital signs of life, the patient has lost all response to the external world and all physiological reflexes are gone. The patient may still have irregular breathing, decreased blood pressure, urine and bowel incontinence, relaxed muscles all over the body, and decerebrate rigidity.

Hand Reflexology and Acupressure

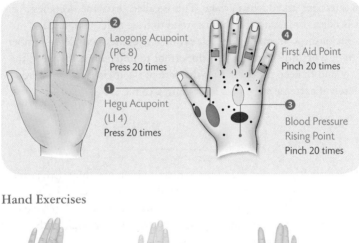

② Laogong Acupoint
(PC 8)
Press 20 times

① Hegu Acupoint
(LI 4)
Press 20 times

④ First Aid Point
Pinch 20 times

③ Blood Pressure
Rising Point
Pinch 20 times

Hand Exercises

① ② ③

1. With your right thumb and index finger, pinch and pull the skin on the back of the little finger along its metacarpal bone until you reach the wrist crease.

2. Use your right thumb and index finger to pinch and pull the skin on the root of the back of the left ring finger

3. Open your palm and spread the fingers out; use a stick to jab the center of the palm in evenly-spread dots.

Other Methods

1. Position the patient's head sideways for easy removal of respiratory secretions. If the patient brings up phlegm, vomit, or other secretions, remove it immediately with suction or manually.

2. Keep the patient's airway unobstructed, and make sure they do

not catch a cold.

3. Patients in a long-term coma usually have a weakened immune system. Prevent them from developing bedsores and any other secondary infections.

4. Please note: Some patients fall asleep very easily, and find it hard to stay awake. However, they can be woken up, and can respond to questions asked when awake. This is called "extreme sleepiness." It is not a coma, and the patients tend to have mildly impaired consciousness. In many diseases, extreme sleepiness and deep slumber can be a prelude to coma. It is important to differentiate between the two, and to keep a close eye on the patient's consciousness. Monitor closely if extreme sleepiness lapses into a coma.

7. Eye Fatigue

When tired, your eyes may hurt and your vision may blur. Eye fatigue may also trigger symptoms such as headache, heaviness of the head, and stiff shoulders. Eye fatigue due to refractive errors and unbalanced eye muscles may cause myopia, astigmatism, or presbyopia with different prescriptions for both eyes.

Primary causes of eye fatigue include:

- Excessive use of the eyes, e.g., staring at the computer screen at work. Prolonged use of the eyes without blinking will make the corneal surface become dry and irritate the cornea.
- Reading in strong and dim lights for prolonged periods of time.
- Wearing the wrong prescription eye glasses, either higher or lower than needed.
- Refractive errors, including myopia, hyperopia, and astigmatism, which are not corrected in a timely manner.
- A severe difference of diopter between the two eyes, e.g., one at -2.00 and the other at -6.00.

Manifestations and Symptoms

Symptoms of eye fatigue include dry eyes, a gritty sensation, heaviness of the eyelids, blurred vision, increased sensitivity to light, watery eyes, bursting pain in the eyes, and redness. In more severe cases, the patient may experience light-headedness, headaches, nausea, lethargy, trouble concentrating, memory problems, poor appetite, and general symptoms such as soreness in the neck, shoulders and back, and numbness of the finger joints.

Hand Reflexology and Acupressure

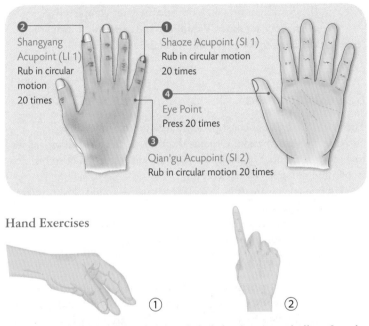

Shangyang Acupoint (LI 1)
Rub in circular motion
20 times

Shaoze Acupoint (SI 1)
Rub in circular motion
20 times

Eye Point
Press 20 times

Qian'gu Acupoint (SI 2)
Rub in circular motion 20 times

Hand Exercises

1. Bend the fingers of your left hand slightly, forming a hollow fist; the tip of the thumb and the tip of the little finger jab against each other.

2. Keep your hand flat with the back against you, and then abruptly withdraw the thumb, the middle finger, the ring finger, and the little finger, leaving only the index finger pointing upward, as if signaling the number "1."

Other Methods

1. People with eye fatigue should develop a healthy lifestyle and good habits to maintain eye health. These include preventing exposure to strong light in particular, and adjusting the brightness of the computer screen to a comfortable level. Give your eyes adequate rest: take a 5- to 10-minute break if your eyes have worked for an hour; do not read or watch TV in a moving vehicle.

2. You can try the following to relieve the symptoms: First, blink your eyes quickly while taking a deep breath. Open and close your eyes quickly as you are breathing out. Second, stare at the tip of your nose while taking a deep breath. When inhaling, look at your own nose tip as if you had a lazy eye, making sure you see the sides of your nose too; when exhaling, return your eyes to the normal state and look at an object in the distance until you have breathed out completely.

3. Increase your intake of Vitamin A and carotene, which are "panacea" to protect your eyes and maintain good eyesight.

8. Constipation

There are two types of constipation: Organic and functional.

Organic constipation: Organic disorders of the internal organs lead to a reduced number of bowel movements and excretion of stools, dry stools, and difficulty with excretion.

Functional constipation: No evident cause is found. The primary causes may include:

- Insufficient intake of food, or food lacking in fiber and water, causing insufficient bowel movement.
- Colon movement disorder is often found in irritable bowel syndrome.
- The habit of resisting the urge to defecate due to fast-paced work and study, a change in work routine and schedule, as well as emotional stress.
- Weak abdominal muscles and pelvic floor disorders can make it hard to empty the bowels.
- Frail elderly people may have trouble with bowel movements due to inadequate exercise, intestinal spasm, or an excessively long colon.

Manifestations and Symptoms

Constipation usually manifests itself as decreased number of bowel movements, which occur only once every 3 to 5 days, or even longer. Sometimes the number of bowel movements remains the same, but the consistency of the stools has changed: Dry and hard stools are difficult to pass. In the meantime, you may suffer from headaches, dizziness, a bloated abdomen, fullness of the stomach, regurgitation, poor appetite and sleep, and irritability and anger.

Hand Reflexology and Acupressure

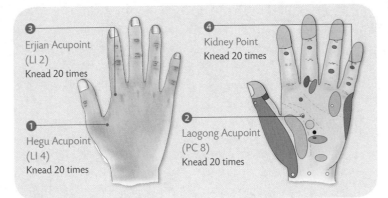

❸ Erjian Acupoint
(LI 2)
Knead 20 times

❶ Hegu Acupoint
(LI 4)
Knead 20 times

❹ Kidney Point
Knead 20 times

❷ Laogong Acupoint
(PC 8)
Knead 20 times

Hand Exercises

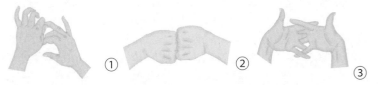

① ② ③

1. Use the thumb and the index finger of one hand to twist and press the ring finger of the other hand in a spiral rotation, starting from the root to the fingertip.

2. Make fists with both hands, palms facing down, and interlock the knuckles of the metacarpal bones so the knuckles press forcefully into the depressions.

3. With palms facing inward, interlock the fingers of both hands; press into and pull away from each other 20 times.

Other Methods

Cultivate a healthy lifestyle and eating habits. A healthy diet will help you to alleviate the pain of constipation. Here are two recommended recipes:

Honey drink: 60 g of honey makes two drinks, 30 g each, for morning and evening daily; dilute the honey in warm water and then drink it. Applicable to the elderly, and to pregnant women.

Honey and royal jelly drink: 60 g honey, 6 g royal jelly; mix them together, and drink with warm water in the morning and the evening every day. Applicable to those suffering from habitual constipation.

Chapter Four

Diseases of the Circulatory and Respiratory Systems

A network of ducts and vessels throughout the human body, the circulatory system includes the cardiovascular and lymphatic systems. The former circulates blood, while the latter circulates lymph fluid. The respiratory system is the general term for the organs that exchange the air inside the body with that of the external world: We breathe out carbon dioxide and breathe in fresh oxygen. The respiratory system consists of respiratory ducts (nasal, larynx and pharynx, trachea and bronchus) and the lungs. This chapter aims to help you improve the health of these two systems.

1. Hypertension

Hypertension, or high blood pressure, is one of the most common diseases in the world, and also one of the biggest risk factors for cardiovascular diseases. It may trigger complications such as myocardial infarction, heart failure, and chronic kidney diseases. The risk of hypertension increases as you age. Women, who have a lower risk of hypertension than males in general, are confronted with a rapidly increasing risk after menopause, which may be even higher than the risk faced by men. In places of higher latitude where it is colder, the prevalence of hypertension is greater than at lower latitudes where it is warmer. Its prevalence at high altitudes is greater than in low altitudes. Hypertension is also related to dietary habits. The more your intake of salt and saturated fat, the higher your blood pressure and the greater the risk of hypertension.

Manifestations and Symptoms

Hypertension has the following symptoms:

Tinnitus: Perception of ringing in both ears, lasting for a prolonged period of time.

Shortness of breath and palpitations: High blood pressure can cause cardiomyopathy, an enlarged heart, and heart failure, which all lead to shortness of breath and palpitations.

Headache: If a patient often has a headache, sometimes severe, accompanied by nausea and vomiting, this could be a sign of hypertension.

Hand Reflexology and Acupressure

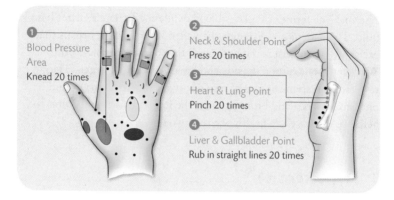

Blood Pressure Area
Knead 20 times

❷ Neck & Shoulder Point
Press 20 times

❸ Heart & Lung Point
Pinch 20 times

❹ Liver & Gallbladder Point
Rub in straight lines 20 times

Hand Exercises

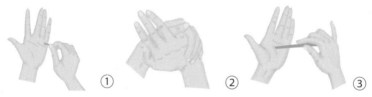

① ② ③

1. Use a stick to jab in evenly-spread dots the transverse creases (creases found when you bend your fingers) of the ring finger with force.

2. With the center of the right palm facing up, withdraw the little finger; your left palm covers your right palm, and presses it while squeezing the little finger of the right hand.

3. Use a pen to jab the center of the palm evenly.

Other Methods

1. Reduce your sodium salt intake. Sodium salt contributes to rising blood pressure, and increases the risk of its occurring. Potassium salt, however, may counteract raised blood pressure caused by sodium salt.

2. Stop smoking. Smoking is one of the major contributing factors to cardiovascular diseases.

3. Limit alcohol intake. Long-term alcohol consumption may lead to hypertension. Reducing your intake can drastically reduce your risk of hypertension.

4. Exercise regularly. Regular physical exercise can reduce blood pressure.

5. Lose weight. Reduced body fat will lower your blood pressure.

6. Reduce emotional stress and keep a balanced state of mind. Negative emotions will increase the risk of cardiovascular disease. Take proactive measures to prevent and reduce your emotional stress. Also, try to correct an unhealthy state of mind, and give it treatment if needed.

2. Hypotension

There is no universal diagnostic standard yet for low blood pressure. In general, an adult is considered to have hypotension if their blood pressure reads below 90/60 mmHg in a limb artery.

Based on the manner of its onset, low blood pressure can either be acute or chronic. Acute low blood pressure refers to a sudden and obvious drop from normal or higher blood pressure, which may be caused by unusual physical weakness. It often happens to young women with very fragile and slender constitutions. Chronic low blood pressure is consistently lower than the normal range.

Manifestations and Symptoms

Symptoms of low blood pressure are faintness, giddiness, feebleness, palpitations, and cognitive impairment. Hypotension often happens in the morning when the affected person gets up from bed. When standing up, they will feel dizziness, weakness in the legs, vertigo, or faintness accompanied by a pale complexion, sweating, nausea, and a change in their pulse rate.

Hand Reflexology and Acupressure

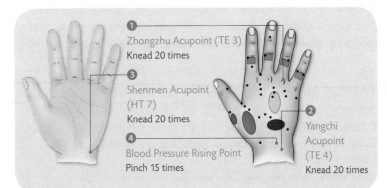

1. Zhongzhu Acupoint (TE 3)
Knead 20 times

3. Shenmen Acupoint (HT 7)
Knead 20 times

4. Blood Pressure Rising Point
Pinch 15 times

2. Yangchi Acupoint (TE 4)
Knead 20 times

Hand Exercises

1. Put a ring on the middle phalanx of the ring finger and turn it to stimulate the finger.

2. Use a toothbrush to brush the palm side of the ring finger back and forth 15 times.

3. Strap a wristwatch on your index finger and last two fingers, and leave your middle finger above the strap.

Other Methods
People with hypotension should maintain a diet that helps to lift the heart and nourish the brain. This includes longan, lotus seeds, dates, and mulberries. Avoid raw and cold food and food that unlock *qi*, such as spinach, radish, and celery, as well as cold drinks and ice cream. Particularly avoid corn, as it tends to reduce blood pressure.

Do more exercise, and improve your overall physical fitness. You can do the following every day: Lie on your back, pull your arms up and interlock your fingers, then make them push and pull against each other for resistance; pull when inhaling; release when exhaling. Repeat this 3 or 4 times, then pull your arms away from the sides of your body to above your head; hold the hands together, and slowly straighten your fingers as you breathe. Then pull back your arms to the sides of your body while inhaling. Repeat as many times as you see fit.

3. Coronary Heart Disease

Coronary atherosclerosis is the primary cause of coronary heart disease. Other factors causing the disease include gender and age, family history, abnormal level of lipids, diabetes, hypertension, smoking, being overweight, obesity, gout, and lack of exercise.

Manifestations and Symptoms

The types of coronary heart disease are as follows:

Angina pectoris: It manifests itself as a squeezing or fullness from behind the chest bones and is often accompanied by anxiety. It lasts 3 to 5 minutes, often emanating to the left side of the hips, shoulders, larynx and pharynx, the back, and the right arm.

Myocardial infarction: Prodrome symptoms often occur a week in advance, such as chest pain while resting or doing light manual labor, accompanied by evident discomfort and fatigue.

Sudden cardiac death: The patient suffers sudden cardiac death as the existing atherosclerosis progresses. When a coronary artery spasm or clog occurs, myocardial infarction will follow, resulting in a local electrophysiological disorder and temporary severe abnormal heart rhythms.

Symptomless myocardial ischemia: Many patients with extensive coronary artery blockage do not feel chest pain. Some may not even experience pain at the time of death.

Hand Reflexology and Acupressure

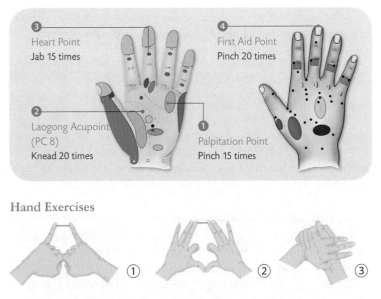

Heart Point
Jab 15 times

First Aid Point
Pinch 20 times

Laogong Acupoint (PC 8)
Knead 20 times

Palpitation Point
Pinch 15 times

Hand Exercises

1. Hold a stick between the tips of your little fingers and press it with the force of the two fingers.

2. Hold a stick with the tips of your middle fingers, while you withdraw the two index fingers and press the thumbs against each other.

3. With your right palm holding on to the left palm, press the withdrawn little finger of the left hand, while the remaining three fingers of the left hand touch and press the back of the right hand.

Other Methods

1. Patients with coronary heart disease should keep warm. Particularly in winter when extreme cold sets in with a strong wind, they should take precautions by wearing a facemask and avoiding walking against the wind. This is because in low temperatures, the heart requires a greater supply of blood, but the contracting coronary artery reduces the supply. As a result, the heart muscle cannot get enough blood, which triggers angina pectoris.

2. Maintain a healthy lifestyle by following a regular daily routine. Go to bed early and get up early, and avoid working late.

3. Keep a balanced diet and eat fresh and light food that are easy to digest. Eat vegetables and fruit to make sure you get enough vitamins.

4. Be active and do exercise based on your ability. Design or select appropriate sports and games to facilitate the circulation of *qi* and blood and alleviate the burden on the heart.

4. Anemia

Anemia is a common clinical condition caused by a decreased number of circulating red blood cells per unit volume. Owing to a variety of causes, anemia is classified as anemia by blood loss, destruction of red blood cells, and decreased or faulty red blood cell production.

Manifestations and Symptoms

Clinically, the patient is described as having pale skin, a lusterless complexion, and rough skin. The patient may have mucocutaneous ulceration as the condition progresses to severity.

Anemia may cause shortness of breath or even trouble breathing when it is severe. Long-time anemia, an excessive workload of the heart, coupled with an insufficient supply of oxygen, may lead to anemic heart disease that manifests as a change of heartbeat accompanied by abnormal heart rhythms and heart failure.

Anemia may also do harm to the nervous system, causing lightheadedness, tinnitus, headache, insomnia, frequent and vivid dreams, memory problems, and an inability to concentrate.

In addition, anemia may cause conditions such as an unusually rapid heartbeat, poor appetite, diarrhea, amenorrhea, and decreased sexual desire. If an infant is anemic, they are susceptible to more crying and irritability. Worse still, it may affect brain development.

Hand Reflexology and Acupressure

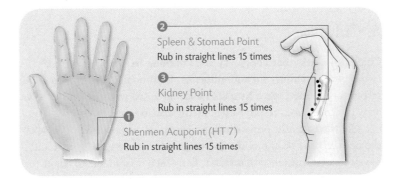

2 Spleen & Stomach Point
Rub in straight lines 15 times

3 Kidney Point
Rub in straight lines 15 times

1 Shenmen Acupoint (HT 7)
Rub in straight lines 15 times

Hand Exercises

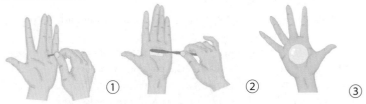

① ② ③

1. Open your palm, spread out the fingers, and use a stick to jab the center of the palm in evenly-spread dots.

2. Use a toothbrush to brush up and down the center of the palm. Repeat 30 times.

3. Place a ball in the center of the palm, spread the fingers, and use the mobility of the roots of the fingers to roll it clockwise and counter-clockwise 10 times respectively.

Other Methods

1. Maintain a balanced diet. Eat regular meals of an appropriate size. Avoid excessive drinking and eating. Choose food of many varieties, and avoid biases in dietary components.

2. Eat food rich in iron, such as pig's liver and blood, lean meat, dairy products, beans, rice, apples, and green vegetables.

3. Drink more tea, which supplements folic acid and vitamin B_{12} and is conducive to the treatment of megaloblastic anemia. However, for those with iron-deficiency anemia, do not drink tea that may hinder the absorption of iron, and eat more acidic food instead.

4. Avoid spicy, raw, and cold food, as they are not easy to digest.

5. Cold

Cold is an illness that goes away after running its course. There are two types: Common cold and influenza. Common cold is a common respiratory illness caused by a cold-causing virus, whereas influenza is an acute contagious respiratory epidemic caused by flu viruses.

Colds are caught primarily because exogenous negative *qi* attacks the body via the skin, mouth, and nose when the system is weak and has decreased resistance to diseases, and when it is unable to adapt to drastic weather changes.

Manifestations and Symptoms

According to TCM, there are three types of cold: wind-cold, wind-heat, and damp-heat.

Wind-cold: In addition to the general symptoms of a stuffy nose, sneezing, coughing, and headache, the patient has an aversion to cold, a low-grade temperature but no sweat, sore muscles, clear and watery nose discharge, thin white phlegm, a painful and swollen throat, absence of thirst or a penchant for hot drinks, and sparse white tongue coating.

Wind-heat: In addition to the general symptoms of a stuffy nose, runny nose, coughing, and headache, the patient runs a high temperature, has thick, sticky yellow phlegm, and a sore throat (usually starting before other cold symptoms); sputum is usually yellow or dark, and the patient may experience constipation.

Damp-heat: Aversion to cold, feverish sensation, no taste in the mouth, headache, distending sensation in the head, abdominal pain, and diarrhea.

Hand Reflexology and Acupressure

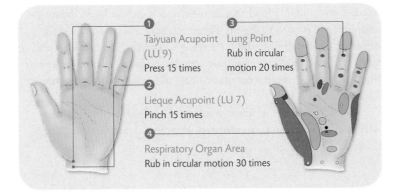

Taiyuan Acupoint (LU 9)
Press 15 times

Lung Point
Rub in circular motion 20 times

Lieque Acupoint (LU 7)
Pinch 15 times

Respiratory Organ Area
Rub in circular motion 30 times

Hand Exercises

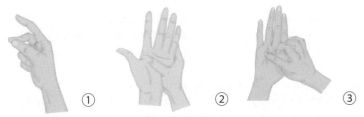

1. Bend the fingers slightly, align your thumb with the middle finger, and press the tips of the two fingers against each other.

2. Use your thumb and the index finger to press and rub the center of the other palm.

3. With your right thumb and index finger, pull and pinch the skin on the back of the ring finger at its root.

Other Methods

1. Tips for cold prevention: Wash hands often, open windows often for fresh air, avoid bodily contact with the affected, take adequate rest, drink plenty of water, and keep a regular daily schedule.

2. In the early stage of cold, use a blow dryer on temples for 3 to 5 minutes a few times daily, to help relieve the symptoms.

3. In addition to getting timely treatment, a balanced diet will help you recuperate. Avoid salty food, which tends to cause the diseased mucous membrane to constrict, thus exacerbating nasal congestion and throat discomfort. Besides, overly salty food can induce more phlegm due to local irritation, and can thus worsen a cough. Avoid sweet and oily food too, as sweetness is conducive to dampness, and oily food is hard to digest. Therefore, stay away from all kinds of candy, sugary drinks, and fatty meat when you have a cold. Avoid spicy food and food containing hot energy, because they are likely to drain your body's fluid, encourage heat, and generate phlegm that is hard to spit out.

4. Soak your feet in warm water for 15 minutes every night, with the water covering your instep. Your feet should turn red after soaking.

6. Pharyngitis

This is an upper respiratory tract disease. Based on the time since its onset and its various symptoms, it can be acute or chronic.

Acute pharyngitis is usually caused by a virus or bacteria. It often happens in winter and spring, and is secondary to acute rhinitis, acute sinusitis, and acute tonsillitis. It is often a complication of contagious diseases such as measles, flu, and scarlet fever.

Chronic pharyngitis is often the result of ineffective treatments of episodes of acute pharyngitis. It can also be the result of other nasal disorders, nasal obstructions, long-term mouth breathing, and irritation of the pharynx due to physical and chemical factors, as well as chemotherapy in the neck.

The illness is often secondary to chronic conditions such as constipation, anemia, cardiovascular disease, and chronic inflammation of the lower respiratory tract.

Manifestations and Symptoms

Primary symptoms are pain and itchiness in the pharynx, trouble swallowing, and a feverish sensation. When compounded with laryngitis, the patient will experience hoarseness of the voice if not severe, and loss of the voice if severe.

Adults mainly suffer symptoms in the pharynx. Early signs include dryness and itchiness, and a burning sensation. It then progresses to pain, which exacerbates when swallowing, excessive secretion of saliva, and ear pain on the inflamed side of the pharynx.

Frail adults or young children may manifest general symptoms such as fever, aversion to cold, headache, poor appetite and sore limbs.

Hand Reflexology and Acupressure

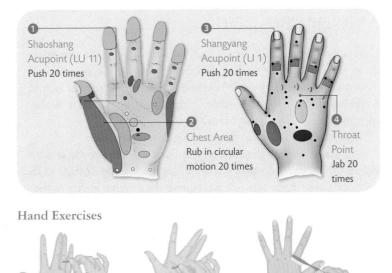

① Shaoshang Acupoint (LU 11) Push 20 times

③ Shangyang Acupoint (LI 1) Push 20 times

② Chest Area Rub in circular motion 20 times

④ Throat Point Jab 20 times

Hand Exercises

① ② ③

1. Use a stick to jab the ring finger in evenly-spread dots, starting from the fingertip downward; at the same time take deep breaths.

2. With the palm facing inward, spread the five digits, and use a stick to jab the transverse creases of the thumb forcefully in evenly spread dots.

3. Brush the Hegu acupoint up and down with a toothbrush.

Other Methods

An appropriate diet may help the patient recuperate:

Congee with *goji* berries: Wash sticky rice and *goji* berries, and then soak them in water for 30 minutes. Cook on gentle heat and simmer until the congee is ready. Eat a bowl of it every day. The congee nourishes *yin* and moistens the throat, and is good for chronic laryngitis and dry throat.

Sugar cane and radish drink: Cook lily bulbs until they are mushy, then mix with sugar cane juice and white radish juice. Drink one glass before going to bed at night. It nourishes *yin* and reduces heat, which is good for voice fatigue and chronic laryngitis.

7. Chronic Bronchitis

Chronic bronchial asthma is a chronic inflammation of the airways, the mucosa around the trachea, and the bronchus and surrounding tissues, usually caused by infection and other physio-chemical factors. A weakened immune system plays an important role in the formation and development of chronic bronchial asthma.

Contributing factors to chronic bronchial asthma are:

Air pollution: Chlorine, nitric oxide, and sulphur dioxide in the air can irritate the mucosa of the bronchus and may do damage to the epithelial tissue of the airways, weakening the filtering ability of the airways.

Smoking: This is the primary trigger of the disease. Irritating smoke causes the constriction of smooth muscle and encourages active glandular secretion, impeding airflow in the airways.

Infection: Respiratory infection is another important factor that can trigger the onset and worsening of asthma.

Manifestations and Symptoms

Clinical manifestations of bronchial asthma are:

- Long-term repeated coughing episodes: Mainly coughing in the morning, but also bouts of coughing and spitting of sputum when sleeping. As the disease progresses, coughing can become perennial.
- Expectoration: Usually a white viscous or serous frothy phlegm, occasionally containing blood.
- Panting: When panting is evident, it is known as asthmatic bronchitis.

The early symptoms of chronic bronchial asthma are not obvious. It often occurs in winter and subsides in spring when the weather is warm; inflammation worsens in the late stages when the symptoms persist regardless of seasonal changes. As the condition progresses, it can trigger complications such as emphysema, pulmonary hypertension, and an enlarged right side of the heart.

Hand Reflexology and Acupressure

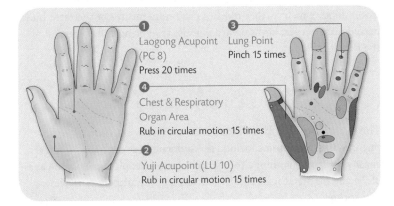

❶ Laogong Acupoint (PC 8)
Press 20 times

❸ Lung Point
Pinch 15 times

❹ Chest & Respiratory Organ Area
Rub in circular motion 15 times

❷ Yuji Acupoint (LU 10)
Rub in circular motion 15 times

Hand Exercises

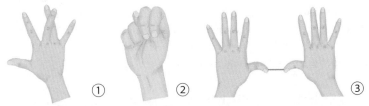

① ② ③

1. Place your palm flat and let your middle finger cross over to hold onto the ring finger. Move from the top down to press the ring finger with force.

2. Tuck your thumb between your middle finger and index finger, and contract the other four fingers with force to press the thumb.

3. Hold a stick with the tips of both thumbs and press it hard with the force of the thumbs.

Other Methods

People with chronic bronchial asthma should follow a good diet to keep healthy:

1. Eat more protein, such as eggs, lean meat, milk, animal liver, fish, and soy products.

2. On days when the temperature is unusually low, eat more food with high calories and warm energy to maintain heat, e.g., meat; also eat plenty of fresh vegetables and fruit to ensure adequate Vitamin C intake.

3. Avoid frozen food and ice cream in summer. Ice crystals (from the water content) are likely to irritate the oral cavity when you eat frozen food, which further reduces the temperatures of the taste buds, periodontal nerves, and salivary glands, triggering inflammation of the throat.

8. Streptococcus Pneumoniae Infection ....

This is an acute alveolar inflammation caused by streptococcus pneumoniae. Symptoms include the sudden onset of chills, high fever, chest pain, and coughing. Young and healthy people between the ages of 20 and 40 are at high risk of contracting it, particularly in winter and spring.

When the body's immune system is normal, streptococcus pneumoniae are regular bacterium in the oral cavity, nose, and throat. Streptococcus pneumoniae infection often happens in winter and early spring. They become toxic when ordinarily healthy people catch cold, are caught in the rain, or are tired or drunk. It also occurs when the immune system is weakened by a viral infection.

Manifestations and Symptoms

This disease usually has premonitory symptoms of upper respiratory tract infection. The onset is sudden, accompanied by high fever, chills, and sore muscles all over the body. The sufferer's temperature can reach as high as 39 to 40 ℃ within a few hours, peaking in the afternoon or early evening, with an acceleration of the pulse. Sufferers typically have flushed cheeks, nasal flaring, dry hot skin, and herpes simplex in the corners of the mouth and around the nose. Some patients may have chest pain on the affected side, which can emanate to the shoulder or abdomen; pain increases as coughing or deeper breathing occur; there is little phlegm, but blood or rust-colored secretions may be seen in it. The patient may also have occasional nausea, abdominal pain or diarrhea, which could lead to misdiagnosis as acute abdomen syndrome.

Hand Reflexology and Acupressure

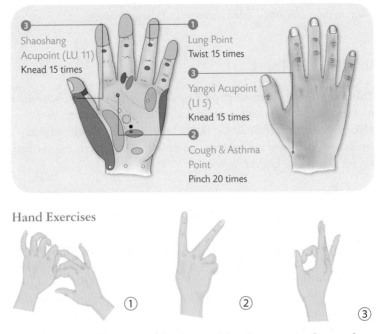

❸ Shaoshang
Acupoint (LU 11)
Knead 15 times

❶ Lung Point
Twist 15 times

❸ Yangxi Acupoint
(LI 5)
Knead 15 times

❷ Cough & Asthma
Point
Pinch 20 times

Hand Exercises

①   ②   ③

1. Use the thumb and index finger of one hand to twist and press the ring finger of the other hand in spiral rotation, starting from the root to the fingertip.

2. Stretch out your index and middle fingers and keep them attached side by side. Then, abruptly move the index finger away to form a "V" sign.

3. Place your palm flat out; bring your middle finger toward the thumb while keeping the index, ring, and little fingers straight.

Other Methods

Follow a healthy diet to promote the results of medical treatment and improve the body's resistance to the disease:

1. Eat plenty of nutritious food that is high in calories and protein, to nourish the body's energy after high fever.

2. An imbalance of acid and alkaline is a common sign of pneumonia. Eat more fresh vegetables and mineral-rich fruit to reverse water and electrolyte disorders.

3. Eat food that is rich in iron, such as meat and egg yolk; eat food rich in copper such as animal liver and sesame paste, as well as high-calcium food like small dried shrimps and dairy products.

9. Tuberculosis

Tuberculosis is an infectious respiratory disease caused by mycobacterium tuberculosis. Most patients contract it through the respiratory system. Mycobacterium tuberculosis can be latent for months in dim and damp environments. When sufferers spit out phlegm, the bacteria can become air-born, infecting healthy people.

Manifestations and Symptoms

The onset is typically slow, but the disease can be long-lasting. The main symptoms include:

Systemic: Systemic toxic symptoms are a low fever in the afternoon (around 37.4 to 38 ℃), which can last for weeks; some patients may have recurring hot flushes on the cheeks, centers of the palms, and soles of the feet. Other symptoms include fatigue, unintentional weight loss, and night sweats.

Respiratory: Dry cough, or a cough with just a little mucus, which is usually white. When there is a secondary infection, the bronchial tract expands and the patient coughs up yellow sputum, with varying degrees of blood in it. When the patient has pleural effusion and pneumothorax, breathing can be difficult.

Hand Reflexology and Acupressure

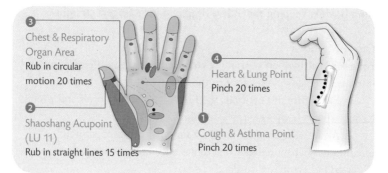

❸ Chest & Respiratory Organ Area
Rub in circular motion 20 times

❹ Heart & Lung Point
Pinch 20 times

❷ Shaoshang Acupoint (LU 11)
Rub in straight lines 15 times

❶ Cough & Asthma Point
Pinch 20 times

Hand Exercises

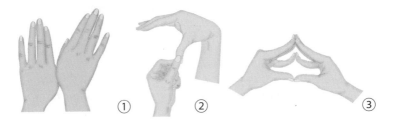

1. With the palms facing down, attach the radial sides of the heels of the palms side by side; withdraw the thumbs and rub the metacarpal sides against each other.

2. With the right palm facing down, use your left thumb and the index finger to pinch the right thumb and pull it vertically downward.

3. Align your fingertips face to face, and press them with force so that they form the biggest possible angle.

Other Methods

Treatment and recuperation from tuberculosis take a long time. The patient should be prepared to fight the disease and maintain good spirits. They should exercise regularly and incrementally to stay physically fit. They should also take good care of themselves, and cooperate with the treatment to ensure a full recovery.

Patients in the advanced stage are usually very fragile and need a higher dietary intake of protein, calories, and fiber to strengthen the immune system. During this period, patients should stay in bed, especially those who are feverish, coughing up blood, or suffering pulmonary insufficiency in the compensatory mechanisms. Those who do not have obvious toxic symptoms can engage in general exercises, but should restrict themselves to a moderate level.

From remission to stabilization, the patient should increase the intensity of exercise, but must not over-exercise to avoid the possibility of a relapse.

Patients with tuberculosis generally have a weakened immune system and should avoid contracting respiratory infections.

10. Bronchial Asthma

Bronchial asthma, also known simply as asthma, is a chronic inflammation of the airway in response to eosinophils and mast cells. This inflammation will trigger varying degrees of reversible airway obstruction.

There are three causes of bronchial asthma: Irritants in the air, infection, and food allergens. Irritants in the air are either specific or non-specific. The former includes pollen, fungus, animal hair, and dander, whereas the latter includes chemicals such as sulphuric acid, sulphur dioxide, and chloramine. The development and onset of asthma is related to repeated infections of the respiratory airway. It is not uncommon that some food may trigger asthma attacks.

Manifestations and Symptoms

Asthma manifests itself as a sudden difficulty breathing, accompanied by wheezing, rapid breathing, and foamy sputum. Inhaling is relatively easy, but exhaling is hard. During an attack, the patient can hear his or her own wheezing. Onsets most often occur at night or early in the morning. Asthma attacks come and go. Most will subside on their own. In some cases, an attack can last 24 hours, resulting in more serious conditions such as cyanosis, when the patient's lips and extremities turn bluish.

Hand Reflexology and Acupressure

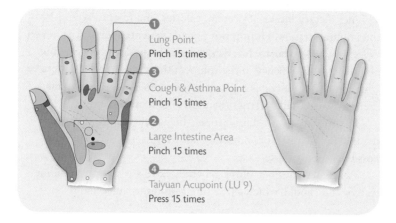

1. Lung Point
Pinch 15 times

3. Cough & Asthma Point
Pinch 15 times

2. Large Intestine Area
Pinch 15 times

4. Taiyuan Acupoint (LU 9)
Press 15 times

Hand Exercises

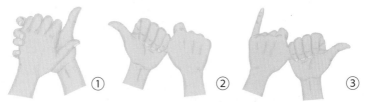

① ② ③

1. Hold your right palm with the left; with your fingers, firmly clasp the back of your other hand, and press and squeeze with force.

2. With the four fingers of the left hand, clasp the thumb of the right hand by its root and pull it outward slowly but forcefully.

3. Wrap the four fingers of the right hand around the left thumb by its root and pull the thumb outward slowly but forcefully.

Other Methods

Do more exercise to improve physical fitness and strengthen the immune system. Stay away from allergens. These measures will help to prevent bronchial asthma attacks.

You should also eat fresh, light food containing plenty of protein and iron.

1. Avoid spicy and irritating food, especially fish, shrimps, and prawns, which are considered likely to trigger asthma.

2. Avoid fatty meat and similar food, as oil tends to generate dampness in the body.

3. Avoid food that generates wind in your body, such as chives and sweet potatoes.

4. Eat more lean meat, animal liver, tofu, and soy milk.

5. Eat plenty of fresh vegetables and fruit. Fresh vegetables not only provide the human body with a variety of vitamins and inorganic salt, but also help to clear phlegm and remove fire; fruit not only helps to clear phlegm and relieve coughing, but also invigorates the spleen and nourishes the lungs.

Chapter Five

Neurological and Endocrine Disorders

M astering the coordination of the physiological functions of the human body, the neurological system mainly consists of the nervous system, including the central nervous system and the peripheral nervous system. The endocrine system also regulates the functions of the body. It includes two categories:

1. The visible organs that exist independently, i.e., endocrine secretion organs such as the pituitary, thyroid, and the adrenal glands.

2. Endocrine organisms and tissues hidden in other organs and tissues across the body, such as islets in the pancreas and follicular cells in the ovaries.

If you perform the hand massage and exercises in this chapter, you will improve the health of your neurological and endocrine systems.

1. Neuralgia

Neuralgia is a pain caused by damaged nerves, which radiates to the nerves it regulates. When the cause is unknown, the disease is called congenital neuralgia; if there is an obvious cause, it is called secondary neuralgia.

Trigeminal neuralgia and sciatica are common forms of neuralgia. Trigeminal neuralgia may be related to factors such as deformed small blood vessels and petrous temporal bones. Sciatica may be caused by tumors in the spinal cord, spinal tuberculosis, lumbar spinal stenosis, pelvic tumors, pressure on the uterus during pregnancy, hip trauma, and diabetes.

Manifestations and Symptoms
Trigeminal neuralgia: Also known as facial neuralgia due to excruciating pain in the cheek, the frontal part of the head, and the forehead. The onset is characterized by a sudden attack of flashing pain that lasts for a few seconds to a few minutes, and an unbearable burning sensation. Episodes of trigeminal neuralgia are of different durations, and pain can be triggered by activities such as washing the face, brushing the teeth, and eating.

Sciatica: The sciatic nerve is the largest nerve in the human body. It starts in the lumbar spine, travels through the pelvis and sciatic foramen to the hip, and then runs along the back of the thigh to the foot. When one raises a heavy object, or squats or rises up too quickly, pain will be triggered from the lower back to the back of the thighs.

Hand Reflexology and Acupressure

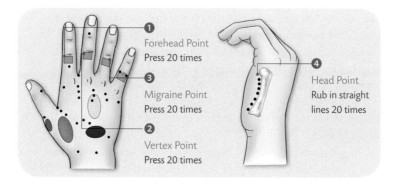

Forehead Point
Press 20 times

Migraine Point
Press 20 times

Vertex Point
Press 20 times

Head Point
Rub in straight
lines 20 times

Hand Exercises

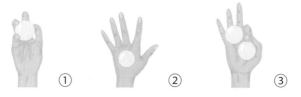

1. Hold a ball with the tips of your five digits; use the mobility of the fingers to turn the ball without touching the center of the palm.

2. Put the ball on the back of your hand and keep it rolling back and forth, left and right.

3. Put two balls in your palm and keep them attached, and then use the mobility of the fingers to turn them.

Other Methods

In everyday life, people with neuralgia should pay attention to the following:

1. Keep a routine of regular daily activities and a balanced diet; get enough sleep and rest; avoid excessive fatigue.

2. Be careful with your movements: Go slowly as much as you can, to avoid triggering potential pain and stimulating sensitive spots.

3. Keep warm when the temperature is low, and avoid exposing your face directly to cold wind.

4. Eat soft food. If pain is triggered by chewing, eat liquid food, and avoid food that is fried, spicy, and irritating; also avoid seafood and the food that are high in heat energy.

2. Neurosis

Neurosis is the result of mental disorders, and can manifest as a variety of mental and physical discomforts. However, examinations are likely to reveal no pathological features in the body.

Although its pathogenesis is related to many fields such as biology, psychology, and sociology, it is mainly caused by mental disorders that occur due to societal factors. When the patient experiences anxiety, stress, mood swings, or psychological trauma, problems will occur in the central nervous system's excitation and inhibition process. The cardiovascular system, which is controlled by the autonomic nervous system, will also malfunction, leading to a series of symptoms associated with excess tension in the sympathetic nervous system.

Manifestations and Symptoms

Cardiac neurosis: This manifests symptoms such as tightness in the chest, palpitations and panting, anxiety, and fright, but examination shows no organic disorders of the heart.

Gastric neurosis: This often manifests as acid reflux, belching, loss of appetite, nausea, vomiting, epigastric burning sensation, fullness and bloating after meals, and discomfort or pain in the upper abdomen, accompanied by fatigue and headache. Gastrointestinal examinations may reveal irritable bowel syndrome or superficial erosive gastritis, but they do not explain the more severe symptoms.

Hand Reflexology and Acupressure

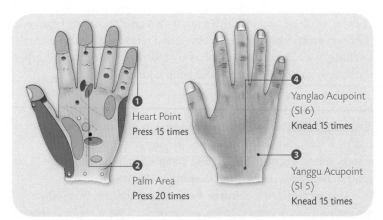

① Heart Point
Press 15 times

② Palm Area
Press 20 times

④ Yanglao Acupoint (SI 6)
Knead 15 times

③ Yanggu Acupoint (SI 5)
Knead 15 times

Hand Exercises

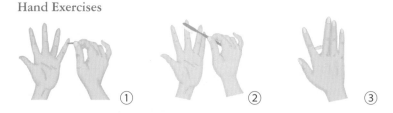

1. Use a stick to jab the little finger evenly from the top down along the phalanx bone line.

2. Use a toothbrush to brush the palm side of the middle finger up and down.

3. Put a coin horizontally between the index finger and the middle finger, and keep it there firmly with the force of the fingers.

Other Methods

An appropriate diet is often complementary to treatment. Lotus seeds and lily bulbs are conducive to nourishing the heart and tranquilizing the mind, and facilitate the treatment of neurosis.

Parents should help their children develop into psychologically healthy people, and should support and encourage them to face challenges so that they foster a personality of resilience, calmness, tenacity, and openness, and an ability to rise to the challenges of life.

3. Epilepsy

Epilepsy is a condition in which a group of highly excitatory neurons in the brain experience sudden, excessive, and repeated electrical events, resulting in a sudden and temporary dysfunction of the brain. Epilepsy is primarily caused by genetics and brain injuries.

Manifestations and Symptoms

Tonic-clonic (grand mal) seizures: Sudden loss of consciousness, and then uncontrollable stiffness and jerking and shaking, often accompanied by screaming, a bluish complexion, loss of bladder control, biting the tongue, and foaming in the mouth.

Absence (petit mal) seizures: Sudden disconnection from others around you, loss of consciousness, accompanied by a myoclonic seizure.

Hand Reflexology and Acupressure

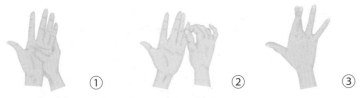

3 Zhongchong
Acupoint (PC 9)
Knead 20 times

2 Guanchong
Acupoint (TE 1)
Knead 20 times

1 Heart Point
Rub in circular
motion 20 times

4 Yanggu
Acupoint (SI 5)
Knead 20 times

Hand Exercises

① ② ③

1. With your thumb and index finger, pinch the center of the other palm and expand in concentric circles.

2. With your thumb and the index finger, pinch the little finger of the other hand in spiral rotation, starting from the root and going upwards.

3. With your palm facing outward, cross your index finger over the back of the middle finger, pressing with as much force as possible.

Other Methods

1. Maintain a light diet; eat more vegetables and fruit; avoid pungent and spicy food and caffeinated drinks such as coffee and coca cola; quit smoking and alcohol.

2. Avoid taking medicines containing caffeine and ephedrine, and medicines such as penicillin or floxacin drugs, which could trigger an onset.

3. Keep a regular life schedule by having a fixed bedtime routine; make sure you have enough sleep, and avoid staying up late or engaging in excessive physical strain; avoid watching TV and playing electronic games for extended periods.

4. People with epilepsy are forbidden from driving and swimming in the sea or rivers. They should not take up occupations that involve aerial work or operating machines.

4. Cranial Nerve Injuries

Cranial nerve injuries include traumatic brain injuries (mostly related to basal skull fractures) and sequelae of cerebral arteriosclerosis (cerebral hemorrhage and cerebral venous sinus thrombosis), sequelae of encephalitis and meningitis, and sequelae of demyelinating disease.

Manifestations and Symptoms
Damage to the olfactory nerves: Damage to the olfactory bulb and olfactory tract, leakage of cerebrospinal fluid, partial or complete loss of olfactory sensation on one side or both sides.

Damage to the visual nerves: Reduced vision or even loss of vision; loss of direct light reflection, with normal indirect light reflection.

Damage to the facial and auditory nerves: Facial palsy at different times, loss of taste capacity by two thirds on the same side of the tongue, keratitis, tinnitus, vertigo, and sensorineural hearing loss.

Hand Reflexology and Acupressure

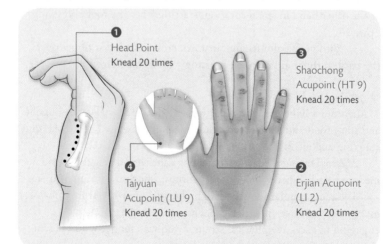

❶ Head Point
Knead 20 times

❸ Shaochong
Acupoint (HT 9)
Knead 20 times

❹ Taiyuan
Acupoint (LU 9)
Knead 20 times

❷ Erjian Acupoint
(LI 2)
Knead 20 times

Hand Exercises

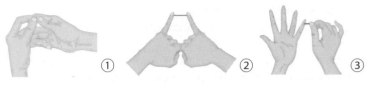

1. Press the tips of two thumbs against each other; bend the remaining fingers and interlock into the fingers of the other hand.

2. Place a stick between the tips of the two little fingers and use the force of the little fingers to press it.

3. Use a stick to evenly jab the little finger top down along the phalanx bones.

Other Method
Some research shows that eating curry can help alleviate cranial nerve damage and improve memory.

5. Bipolar Disorder

Bipolar disorder is a common mental illness involving abnormally elevated moods and periodical depression. Sufferers experience much stronger mood swings than others, which last for a long time and can affect social lives and physiological functions.

The exact cause of bipolar disorder is still unknown. In addition to factors such as genetics, extreme mental stress, traumatic events, changes in neurotransmitter function, and neuroendocrine disorders, fast-paced work and strained inter-personal relations are also important factors. Stressful and traumatic events in adverse environment may be triggers. Current studies tend to believe that genetics and environmental factors play an important role in the onset of the disease. By comparison, genetic factor may play a more prominent role.

Manifestations and Symptoms
The onset of this disease includes two modes: mania/hypomania and depression. As for its manifestations, the affected can either be exceptionally elated, happy, worry-free, and in high spirits, or depressed, sad, melancholy, sullen, unpleasant, lacking confidence, or even hopeless about the future; worse still, the affected may inflict pain

on themselves and be susceptible to suicidal thoughts and behaviors.

Some patients may flare into a rage due to trifling matters or irritability. Some may engage in provocative behavior if seriously irritated.

Patients alternating between the two modes are bi-directional, whereas those who suffer only one form are one directional.

Hand Reflexology and Acupressure

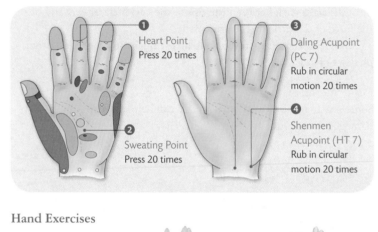

Heart Point
Press 20 times

Daling Acupoint
(PC 7)
Rub in circular
motion 20 times

Sweating Point
Press 20 times

Shenmen
Acupoint (HT 7)
Rub in circular
motion 20 times

Hand Exercises

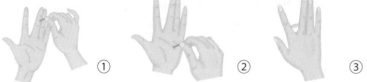

1. Use a stick to jab the palm side of the middle finger in even dots, starting from the fingertip downward.

2. Spread the five digits; use a stick to jab with force along the transverse palmar creases.

3. Put a coin horizontally between the proximal phalanges of the index finger and the middle finger, and keep it there firmly with the force of the fingers.

Other Methods

Maintain a healthy mentality and a good diet; avoid pungent and spicy food. Wheat seedling tea and fungus-tofu soup are good for alleviating the symptoms.

Wheat Seedling Tea: Appropriate amount of green wheat seedlings, orange peel (15 g), field sow-thistle herbs (9 g), 10 dates; cook all ingredients together. Strain and keep the juice. Add some sugar, and drink warm.

Fungus-Tofu Soup: Fungus (30 g), tofu (3 pieces), walnuts (7 pieces). Cook in water, drink the soup, and eat the contents.

6. Acute Cerebrovascular Disease

Acute cerebrovascular disease is one of the three most common causes of death, and refers to a group of events that hinder cerebrovascular blood circulation. The onset is usually abrupt. The underlying causes may vary, from abrupt cerebral thrombosis, cerebral ischemic stroke, or cerebral hemorrhagic stroke due to cerebrovascular rupture. Hemorrhagic cerebrovascular disease is a result of hypertension, cerebral atherosclerosis, congenital cerebral aneurysm, and cerebrovascular deformity.

Manifestations and Symptoms
Dizziness, headache, blurred vision, hemiplegia, and uncontrollable shaking. If the condition is severe, the patient may suffer loss of vision, vertigo, vomiting, and quadriplegia.

Hand Reflexology and Acupressure

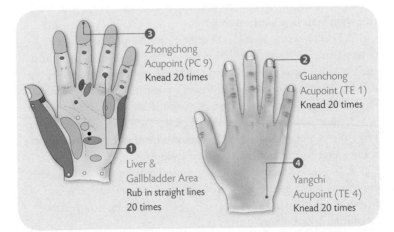

Zhongchong
Acupoint (PC 9)
Knead 20 times

Guanchong
Acupoint (TE 1)
Knead 20 times

Liver &
Gallbladder Area
Rub in straight lines
20 times

Yangchi
Acupoint (TE 4)
Knead 20 times

Hand Exercises

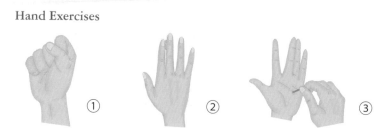

1. Open your palm, and quickly fold in the four fingers, with the thumb tightly attached.

2. With your palm facing outward, tuck a coin between the index and middle fingers and keep it there firmly; make the coin move up and down slightly without falling out.

3. Spread the five digits. Use a stick to jab with force along the transverse palmar creases from the top down.

Other Methods

1. Lifestyle: Avoid staying in bed for too long, as it will reduce blood circulation, which can lead to ischemic stroke, and is not conducive to poststroke physiological recuperation; when temperatures are low, put on a few more layers of clothes to stay warm, and wear gloves, a hat, a scarf, and an overcoat when going out. This will help prevent blood vessels contraction causing hypertension and exacerbate your condition. Do not take off your quilt as soon as you wake up, and make sure the room is warm (ask a family member to turn the heating on) before you get up; heat the bathroom before going in to wash; brush your teeth and wash your face with warm water.

2. Diet: Increase your intake of highprotein food such as fish, poultry, and lean meat; avoid food that is rich in saturated fatty acid such as fatty meat, animal fat, and offal; control your salt intake, but if using dehydrating agent or diuretics, properly increase the amount; ensure that you eat plenty of vitamins and fresh vegetables every day.

3. Mental health: Maintain good control of your emotions and stay calm; avoid excessive fatigue, and shun extreme emotions such as ecstasy, rage, depression, sorrow, fear, and fright.

4. General: Keep risk factors in control; have a physical checkup once every six or twelve months; do not replace medication with health supplements; do not stop taking lipidlowering drugs without consulting your doctor.

7. Diabetes

Diabetes is a common endocrine and metabolic disorder. Its main causes are:

• Deficiency of the immune system: A number of immune antibodies are found in the blood of people with diabetes. These abnormal antibodies may damage β-cells, which help to produce insulin from the pancreas.

• Genes: Current research points to genetic deficiency as the basic cause of diabetes.

• Viral infections: Diabetes may be triggered by a virus. Sufferers are often found to have been infected with a virus before the onset.

Manifestations and Symptoms
Clinical diagnosis is based on the indicator of high glucose; common symptoms are excessive thirst and hunger, frequent urination, and weight loss.

Some patients with Type II diabetes may not have any symptoms apart from dizziness and feebleness. Early diabetes or pre-diabetes may manifest as low glucose before lunch or dinner.

Hand Reflexology and Acupressure

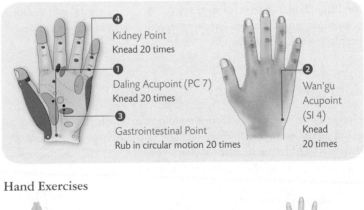

4 Kidney Point
Knead 20 times

1 Daling Acupoint (PC 7)
Knead 20 times

3 Gastrointestinal Point
Rub in circular motion 20 times

2 Wan'gu Acupoint (SI 4)
Knead 20 times

Hand Exercises

①

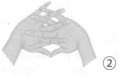
②

③

1. With the palms facing each other, bend the index finger and the middle finger over, leaving the ring finger and the little fingers pressing against each other while moving left and right.

2. With the palms leaning towards each other sideways, interlock the fingers; press them against each other, and push them away from you.

3. With the right palm facing down, lock the fingers of the left hand into the right hand from the back, and press as hard as you want.

Other Methods

Dietary changes may prove to be the most important factor in treating diabetes. The general principle is to control weight and calorie intake.

1. Reduce fat in your food, particularly saturated fatty acid; increase your intake of fiber, and keep an appropriate proportion of carbohydrates, fats, and proteins in your diet.

2. Control your overall calorie intake, balance your nutrition, and maintain a healthy weight.

3. Eat less: take the initiative in controlling the amount of food you eat; eat appropriate portions; eat more whole grains.

4. More exercise: do exercise every day, particularly for aerobic metabolism; practice massage every day.

When doing exercise outside the home, take some sweets with you. Eat one if you feel light-headed. Prepare a health information card about yourself, including information such as your name and health condition, home address, emergency contact, the hospital and doctor you usually go to. This way, if an emergency occurs (such as fainting) people around you will be able to help.

8. Hyperthyroidism

Hyperthyroidism is an endocrine condition in which your thyroid gland produces too much thyroxin. The causes of hyperthyroidism are closely related to the immune system, genetics, and the environment, e.g., trauma, traumatic experiences, and infection.

Manifestations and Symptoms

Manifestations in metabolic syndrome patients include increased appetite, weight loss, aversion to heat, palpitations, and excitement. They also include increased excitement of the nerves and blood vessels, as well as varying degrees of such features as enlarged thyroid glands and bulging eyes, shaking hands, and vascular bruit in the neck. If the disease is severe, the patient may experience thyroid crisis, coma, or even death. Senile hyperthyroidism does not usually show these typical signs, but often manifests as apathy, loss of appetite, and obvious weight loss, which can sometimes be misdiagnosed as cancer.

Hand Reflexology and Acupressure

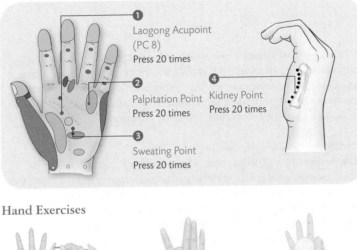

Laogong Acupoint
(PC 8)
Press 20 times

Palpitation Point
Press 20 times

Kidney Point
Press 20 times

Sweating Point
Press 20 times

Hand Exercises

1. Use a stick to poke the little finger evenly along the metacarpal bone from the tip downward.

2. Place a coin horizontally between the roots of the index and the middle fingers, and hold it there firmly with the force of the fingers.

3. Place two balls in your palm, and keep them attached. Then, use the mobility of your fingers to turn the two balls.

Other Methods

Early stage hyperthyroidism should be treated as quickly as possible. Learn about the condition, and take measures to prevent complications and bring the disease under control.

In the early recuperation period, special care should be taken with diet and medication. Regular checkups are necessary. The patient should keep track of their condition and prevent it from reoccurring:

1. Keep a pleasant mood and be free of anxieties in daily life.

2. Maintain an appropriate diet. Avoid pungent and spicy food such as chili pepper, raw green onion, and raw garlic. Avoid seafood such as kelp, sea prawns/shrimps, and ribbonfish.

3. Follow an appropriate daily schedule; strengthen your immune system and your ability to resist disease.

9. Menopause Syndrome

When a woman's ovaries lose their function, she will experience menopause, i.e., turning from childbearing age to non-childbearing age. During this time, women may experience a variety of symptoms due to ovarian dysfunction, hyperpituitarism, and over-secretion of sex hormones, causing autonomic system dysfunction.

Manifestations and Symptoms

Hot flushes on the cheeks, neck, chest, and back; accelerated pulse, mood swings, excitability, difficulty concentrating, paranoia, tension or depression, irritability, insomnia and dreamful sleep, headaches, pain in the lower back and legs, dizziness and tinnitus, swings in blood pressure, frequent urination, urinary incontinence, osteoporosis, back pain, susceptibility to bone fractures; the reproductive organs and breasts may sag in varying degrees. Other symptoms include lengthening of the menstrual period and less menstrual discharge; shortened menstrual cycles and increased period discharge; irregular cycles, length of periods, and discharge; or sudden termination of periods.

Hand Reflexology and Acupressure

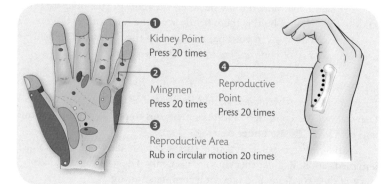

❶ Kidney Point
Press 20 times

❷ Mingmen
Press 20 times

❸ Reproductive Area
Rub in circular motion 20 times

❹ Reproductive Point
Press 20 times

Hand Exercises

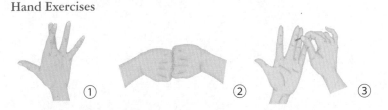

1. Cross your index finger over the middle finger, and press the middle finger down with as much force as possible.

2. Form two fists with the palms facing down; interlock the knuckles of the metacarpal bones so they press into the depressions of the other fist, and press hard.

3. Use a stick to poke the middle finger evenly, from the fingertip downward.

Other Methods

Usually, women suffering from menopausal syndrome do not need special treatment. If they take some measures in daily life regarding their diet, the phase will pass naturally. Men can also experience hormonal changes, but the symptoms are much less obvious, including memory failure, trouble concentrating, loss of sleep, depression, anxiety, irritability, paranoia, and neurosis. To determine if you are suffering from menopause syndrome, go to the hospital for a physical checkup in order to exclude other disease factors. This will include a hormone test, a blood test, and medical imaging for diagnostic determination.

As for diet, sufferers are encouraged to eat food that calms the mind and relieves dryness.

Lotus seed and lily bulb congee: Cook lotus seeds, lily bulbs, and short grain rice together (30 g of each). Eat in the morning and afternoon. This recipe is good for those who suffer palpitations, sleeplessness, forgetfulness, physical fatigue, and rough skin.

Licorice and wheat drink: Cook wheat (30 g), 10 dates, and licorice (10 g) together. Drink the tea once in the morning and once in the afternoon. This is good for those suffering from hot flushes, sweating, irritability, palpitations, depression, ill temper, and lusterless complexion around menopause.

Chapter Six

Diseases of
the Digestive System

The digestive system consists of the digestive tract and digestive glands. The digestive tract includes the mouth, pharynx, esophagus, stomach, small intestine, and large intestine. It also includes auxiliary organs such as the pancreas, liver, and gallbladder. The system ingests, transports, and breaks down food into smaller components so nutrition can be absorbed into the body. Waste from digestion is ejected from the body through defecation. Therefore, the system is of vital importance. A healthy digestive system is related to diet, and promotes a sense of happiness. In this chapter, hand reflexology will assist you in alleviating the symptoms of digestive discomfort and improving the health of your digestive system.

1. Chronic Gastritis

Chronic gastritis is a long-term inflammation of the stomach's mucosa caused by a variety of diseases. It may be triggered or worsened by long-term and excessive alcohol consumption and smoking, irregular eating habits, ingesting food that is too cold, too hot, too coarse, or too hard, and drinking strong tea and coffee. Chronic gastritis is hard to cure when the mucosa is infected by helicobacter pylori.

Manifestations and Symptoms
Many patients have no obvious symptoms. A common symptom is discomfort or pain in the upper abdomen after a meal, or irregular, intermittent, or constant pain in the upper abdomen. If necessary, the patient may undergo a gastric biopsy with gastroscopy to determine whether there is inflammation.

Hand Reflexology and Acupressure

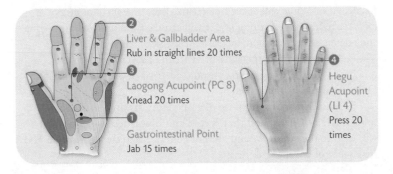

Liver & Gallbladder Area
Rub in straight lines 20 times

Laogong Acupoint (PC 8)
Knead 20 times

Gastrointestinal Point
Jab 15 times

Hegu
Acupoint
(LI 4)
Press 20
times

Hand Exercises

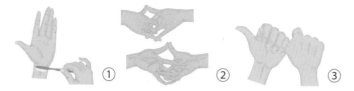

1. Brush the arm side of your wrist crease to the left and right with a toothbrush 30 times.

2. Press your thumbs against each other; hold onto the left middle finger with your right index finger; hold onto the left ring finger with your right middle finger, and press your right little finger against the left little finger.

3. Wrap the four fingers of your left hand around your right thumb by the root, and pull it away forcefully but slowly.

Other Methods

Those suffering from chronic gastritis should maintain a healthy lifestyle and good eating habits:

1. Maintain a controlled diet, avoiding overeating and irregular meal schedules.

2. Be vigilant about food hygiene; make sure external microorganisms cannot attack your mucosa.

3. Try to eat food that is refined, easy to digest, and nutritious.

4. Stay psychologically healthy, because depression, extreme tension, and fatigue can result in the dysfunction of pyloric sphincter, causing bile reflux that eventually leads to chronic gastritis.

The following measures should be taken to prevent chronic gastritis:

1. Avoid smoking and alcohol. Harmful chemicals in tobacco will stimulate the secretion of gastric acid, which erodes the mucosa. Excessive smoking will cause bile reflux. Excessive alcohol intake or long-term drinking of strong liquor will cause gastric mucosal congestion and edema, or even erosion, increasing the risk of chronic gastritis.

2. Medicine abuse (because of other diseases) may harm the mucosa, eventually triggering chronic gastritis or gastric ulceration. Only use drugs as prescribed.

3. Maintain an appropriate diet, avoiding strongly acidic and spicy food, as well as food that is cold and raw. These types of food will irritate the stomach, and are not conducive to the prevention and treatment of chronic gastritis.

2. Gastroptosis

Gastroptosis is the downward displacement of the stomach below the normal range, usually around or even below the iliac crest. The disease is caused by a deficiency in diaphragm suspension, or by the declining function and loosening of the gastrohepatic and gastrocolic ligaments, a decline in intra-abdominal pressure, and abdominal muscle relaxation. Coupled with the patient's constitution and build, the stomach drops down in the shape of an open fishhook. This is what is referred to as "tensionless stomach" in the case of gastroptosis.

Manifestations and Symptoms

Those affected with slight downward displacement may not experience any symptoms.

Those affected with more evident downward displacement may experience discomfort and fullness in the upper abdomen. Symptoms after meals include burping and belching, anorexia, and constipation. Sometimes the patient will feel a dull pain deep in the stomach, which is exacerbated after meal, when standing up, and when tired.

Those affected with the condition in the long term may suffer weight loss, feebleness, and palpitations, as well as perpetual constipation. The unpleasantness of many of the symptoms may lead to mental stress, which causes insomnia, headaches, dizziness, apathy, and depression.

Hand Reflexology and Acupressure

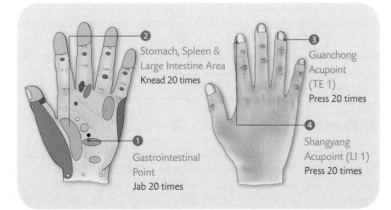

❷ Stomach, Spleen & Large Intestine Area
Knead 20 times

❸ Guanchong Acupoint (TE 1)
Press 20 times

❶ Gastrointestinal Point
Jab 20 times

❹ Shangyang Acupoint (LI 1)
Press 20 times

Hand Exercises

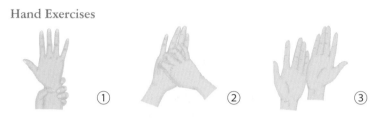

1. With your right palm stretched out facing against you, hold your right wrist in place with your left hand; then, turn your right palm clockwise and counter-clockwise 10 times respectively.

2. With your right thumb and index finger, pinch the skin along the metacarpal bone of the little finger until you reach the wrist crease.

3. With your palms facing up, press the heels of the palms against each other, and rub up and down; repeat it as many times as you want.

Other Methods

The key to the treatment of gastroptosis is to enhance your physical fitness, improve the nutritional components in your diet, and do more exercise that uses the abdominal muscles.

Develop healthy dietary habits: Eat smaller portions but more often, 4 to 6 times a day; chew carefully before swallowing to stimulate gastric movement and accelerate the gastric emptying rate, thus alleviating abdominal discomfort. Reduce the intake of spicy and irritating food, e.g., chili peppers and ginger. Limit your consumption of alcohol and coffee; maintain a balanced food intake of various nutrients.

Exercises: Practice *qigong* and medical exercises, accompanied by walking, jogging, massage, and *taiji*. When practicing *qigong*, lie on your back in bed. Movements should be gentle and slow, with relaxed muscles, and should take place in a quiet ambiance. *qigong* can improve the overall health of the body. It can also increase primordial *qi* in the spleen and stomach, promote gastrointestinal movements, and benefit digestion and absorption, resulting in increased appetite.

3. Peptic Ulcer

A peptic ulcer is a chronic ulceration of the digestive tract and tissues by gastric juice, which contains acid and pepsin. Clinical research has found that over-secretion of gastric acid, helicobacter pylori infection, and the declining protective ability of mucosa are primary factors.

Manifestations and Symptoms

The main features of peptic ulcers are:

1. Chronic, cyclic, and rhythmic onset of upper and middle abdominal pain; an onset typically happens 1 to 2 hours after meal and lasts 1 to 2 hours. The pain subsides when the stomach is empty.

2. A duodenal ulcer often happens on an empty stomach. The symptoms are exacerbated after meals.

3. Other gastrointestinal symptoms include increased secretion of saliva, heartburn, gastric reflux, acid reflux, belching, nausea, and vomiting.

4. Even if a normal appetite is maintained, fear of pain may lead to reduced food intake, causing weight loss.

5. Systemic symptoms may include neurosis such as insomnia, a slow pulse, and excessive sweating.

Hand Reflexology and Acupressure

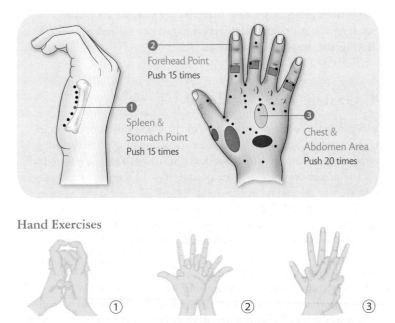

Hand Exercises

1. Press your index fingers and the thumbs against each other at the tip, and interlock the remaining fingers. Press the palms against each other with equal force to create strong resistance.

2. With your left palm facing up, spread the fingers out; interlock your right hand with the fingers of the left hand from behind, and use

the force of the fingers to pinch and press the left hand.

3. With your right palm facing down, lock the fingers of the left hand into those of the right hand from the back whichever way you want, and press with force.

Other Methods
Good care should be taken in daily life:

1. Mental health: Ulcers are more likely to develop if you are experiencing stress, depression, anxiety, or traumatic events. Therefore, having a positive attitude to life is key to the prevention of peptic ulcers.

2. Avoid excessive fatigue: Excessive fatigue will hinder the supply of gastrointestinal blood. Over-secretion of acid and decreased secretion of mucus may damage the mucosa and result in peptic ulcers.

3. Avoid excessive drinking and smoking: Alcohol can be harmful to the protective wall of the gastric mucosa, and may trigger cirrhosis and chronic pancreatitis, thus exacerbating stomach conditions. Smoking can stimulate the secretion of gastric acid and pepsin, which deepens the damage to the mucosa.

4. Gastric and Duodenal Ulcers

It is generally believed that spasms of the blood vessels and muscles of the stomach and duodenum cause the lining of the gastric and duodenum walls to receive inadequate nutrition. This leads to reduced resistance against erosion of the gastrointestinal mucosa by gastric juices.

Healthy people have strong gastrointestinal mucosa that can ward off erosion by gastric acid and pepsin, but when problems occur in any part of the whole chain, ulceration will develop.

Manifestations and Symptoms
Tarry stools and hematemesis (spitting blood): Spitting blood often signals gastric tract bleeding above the duodenum, but tarry stools can be a result of bleeding anywhere in the gastric tract. Spitting blood is invariably accompanied by tarry stools.

Shock: Excessive blood loss will result in shock, a pale complexion, and thirst.

Anemia: Heavy bleeding will lead to reduced counts of hemoglobin, red blood cells, and hematocrit.

Hand Reflexology and Acupressure

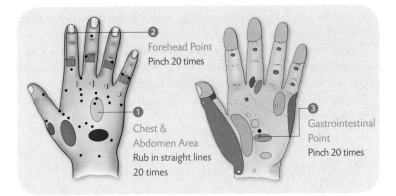

Forehead Point
Pinch 20 times

Chest &
Abdomen Area
Rub in straight lines
20 times

Gastrointestinal
Point
Pinch 20 times

Hand Exercises

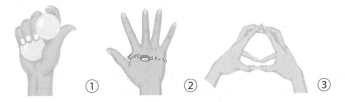

1. Place two balls in your palm, and use the mobility of your fingers to turn them, keeping them apart.

2. Strap a wristwatch or an elastic band on your palm, and stretch your hand so the strap of the watch or the elastic band will stretch or contract as your hand does.

3. With your palms facing each other, press the tips of the five digits to form a hollow ball. Press the tips of the fingers against each other with force.

Other Methods

Daily care for those suffering from gastric and duodenal ulcers involves the following:

1. Healthy cooking: Healthy cooking methods include steaming, boiling, pan-frying, and stewing. Eat lightly, with ginger and pepper to warm the stomach and help protect the mucosa. Food prepared by deep-frying, frying, and smoking are not as digestible, and will impede the healing of the ulcer.

2. Avoid spicy and irritating food, including food that stimulates the secretion of gastric acid, e.g., meat soup, raw green onion, raw garlic, coffee, alcohol, and strong tea, or frozen and extremely hot food, which will irritate the ulcers and worsen the condition.

3. Maintain a nutritious diet with varied ingredients that are easy to digest, and rich in protein, calories, and vitamins. Also, vitamin-rich vegetables and fruit will help expedite the healing of ulcers.

4. Eat food that lubricates the bowels, such as honey, oats, and celery, to prevent dry stools.

5. Calculus of Gallbladder

Calculus of the gallbladder, also known as gallstones, refers to hardened deposits within the bile ducts, and is one of the most common diseases of the digestive system. Clinical manifestations include sudden and rapidly intensifying pain in the abdomen, and acute inflammation.

Manifestations and Symptoms

Early gallstones do not usually have any symptoms. Most are detected through normal physical examination. Sometimes people with gallstones may feel slight discomfort that may be mistaken for gastric disease and not treated in a timely manner.

Some people develop only one stone, while others may have multiple. Sometimes, stones exist freely in the gallbladder. They do not lodge in any specific location, and have no symptoms, hence being called symptomless gallstones.

Small stones may be lodged at the neck of the gallbladder. Symptoms may worsen when one eats oily food that causes the organ to constrict, or when one changes position during sleep. When the gallstone is stuck in the neck of the gallbladder blocking the duct, pressure will grow. Bile cannot be emptied through the neck and duct, leading to a clinical symptom known as biliary colic, which manifests as continued and rapidly intensifying pain in the upper right abdomen, accompanied by nausea and vomiting. If the stone is stuck somewhere and stops moving, the gallbladder can swell and become infected, which will eventually progress to acute cholecystitis.

Hand Reflexology and Acupressure

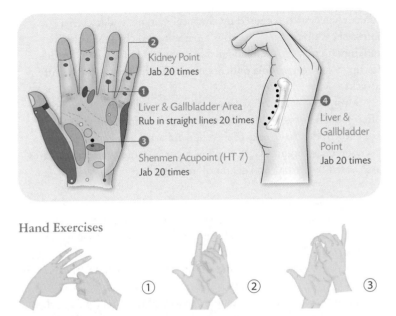

Kidney Point
Jab 20 times

Liver & Gallbladder Area
Rub in straight lines 20 times

Shenmen Acupoint (HT 7)
Jab 20 times

Liver &
Gallbladder
Point
Jab 20 times

Hand Exercises

① ② ③

1. With your right index finger and middle finger, clutch the left index finger by its root and pull away slowly but forcefully.

2. With the thumb and index finger of one hand, pinch and press the root of the index finger of the other where the metacarpal bone meets the index finger.

3. With the thumb and index finger of one hand, pinch and press the tip of the index finger of the other hand.

Other Methods

Those affected with gallstones should maintain a healthy lifestyle and dietary habits:

1. Eat meals at regular times to help evacuate old bile and secrete new.

2. Maintain a varied diet including both meat and vegetables, a good proportion of refined grains, and coarse food grains; food intake should also comply with your physical characteristics; eat more fresh vegetables and fruit, and reduce the intake of high-calorie food.

3. Avoid crash diets.

4. Engage in sporting activities to strengthen the functions of your internal organs and prevent bile stasis.

6. Cholecystitis

Acute cholecystitis is caused by chemical irritants and bacterial infection. Chronic cholecystitis is a pathological change in chronic inflammation of the gallbladder that comes and goes, often lasting for up to ten years. Some patients may suffer biliary colic and acute attacks.

Most cases of cholecystitis are caused by gallstones, a condition often found in obese and middle-aged women. Some patients are affected due to attacks of E. coli, aerobacter aerogenes, and pseudomonas aeruginosa. A small number of acute cholecystitis cases are caused by trauma and chemical irritants.

Manifestations and Symptoms

Acute cholecystitis: Patients primarily experience sudden upper-right abdomen pain, fever, chills, nausea, and vomiting; some also experience jaundice and even shock.

Chronic cholecystitis: Clinical signs are not evident except for abdominal fullness of varying degrees, discomfort in the upper abdomen or upper-right abdomen, constant dull pain or pain in the right shoulder blade, and symptoms of indigestion such as heartburn, burping and belching, and acid reflux. The symptoms may be exacerbated after eating oily food.

Hand Reflexology and Acupressure

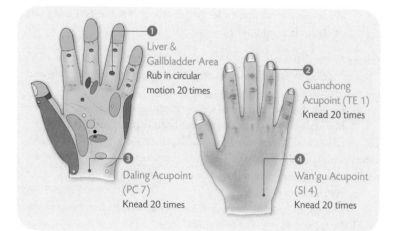

1 Liver & Gallbladder Area
Rub in circular motion 20 times

2 Guanchong Acupoint (TE 1)
Knead 20 times

3 Daling Acupoint (PC 7)
Knead 20 times

4 Wan'gu Acupoint (SI 4)
Knead 20 times

Hand Exercises

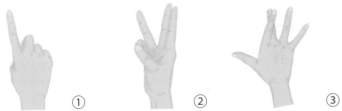

① ② ③

1. With your palm facing outward, abruptly withdraw the thumb and the middle, ring, and little fingers, leaving only the index finger, as if signaling the number "1."

2. Straighten the index and the middle fingers to form a finger-counting sign for the number "2" (Note: all other fingers bend inward, as in a fist) and then quickly stretch out the ring finger. Repeat 10 times.

3. Cross your index finger over the middle finger, and press the middle finger down with as much force as you can.

Other Methods

A healthy lifestyle will help prevent the condition from deteriorating, and will improve your overall physical fitness:

1. Rich intake of vitamins, particularly Vitamins A, C, and E.

2. Appropriate intake of dietary fiber to stimulate intestinal movement and prevent the onset of cholecystitis.

3. Eat small portions often, which will stimulate the contraction of the gallbladder to empty bile and promote its flow.

4. Healthy cooking methods, such as boiling, roasting, steaming, blanching, braising, and stewing; avoid high-temperature stir-frying, deep frying, or frying, as hot oil is likely to irritate the bile duct, causing acute spasms.

5. Fasting is recommended when the patient is experiencing acute biliary colic, but an IV injection can be given as a nutritional supplement.

7. Enteritis

Enteritis is divided into two kinds according to the course of the illness: Acute and chronic.

Shigella is the most common bacteria that causes enteritis. Other factors include eating inedible items, contaminated or stale food, chemical irritants, exposure to toxic amounts of heavy metals, as well as some allergies and the overuse of antibiotics.

Manifestations and Symptoms

Digestive tract symptoms: Nausea, vomiting, abdominal pain, and diarrhea are the main symptoms.

Systemic symptoms: Usually not obvious, but if it is more serious, the patient may experience fever, dehydration, acid poisoning, and shock.

Physical signs: None in the early stage, or if the disease is not serious. The patient may experience slight pain when pressing the upper abdomen or around the belly button, with progressive gurgling sounds. The course of the disease for an average patient is usually short, and cases will clear up on their own within a few days.

Hand Reflexology and Acupressure

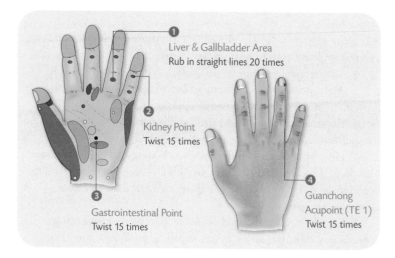

Liver & Gallbladder Area
Rub in straight lines 20 times

Kidney Point
Twist 15 times

Gastrointestinal Point
Twist 15 times

Guanchong Acupoint (TE 1)
Twist 15 times

Hand Exercises

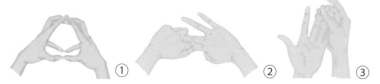

① ② ③

1. With your palms facing each other, press the tips of all the fingers against each other to form a hollow ball.

2. Use the middle and index fingers of the left hand to clutch the middle finger of your right hand. Pull away slowly and forcefully.

3. With your right thumb and middle finger, pinch and twist the left middle finger in spiral rotation.

Other Methods

Patients should pay attention to the following:

1. Maintain a diet that is low in oil and fiber, and eat only light fluid food at the onset of the disease.

2. When the number of bowel movements decreases, stay on a full liquid diet such as meat soup, milk, soy milk, and egg soup. Then, move on to a light semi-fluid diet.

3. When diarrhea stops completely, add soft food such as egg custard, slices of fish, ground lean meat, and vegetable paste. Control the total amount of food you eat every day to avoid indigestion.

As the condition improves, the patient may start a course of food therapy to aid recuperation:

Coix Seed Congee: Coix seeds and short grain rice (30 g to 50 g each) and some sugar. Wash the coix seeds and short grain rice clean. Add water to the mixture and cook until tender; then add some sugar. After the sugar melts, it is ready to eat.

Lotus Seed Congee: Lotus seeds and short grain rice (30 g each), roasted lentils (10 g), 10 small dates, and some sugar. Wash the rice, put all the ingredients together, and cook them. When it is done, add sugar and eat.

8. Hemorrhoids

Hemorrhoids are clusters of varicose veins at the end of the rectum and anal canal. The condition is often found in adults. Due to the varying locations of the growths, hemorrhoids are classified as external, internal, and mixed.

They have many causes.

Anatomical reasons: When a person stands or sits, the rectum and the anus are pulled by gravitational force and the pressure from the organs. This makes the upward flow of blood in the veins difficult, and therefore blood vessels may expand due to blood stagnation.

Occupational reasons: Some people often stand or sit for a long time, or carry heavy objects for long trips. This hinders the flow of blood back to the heart, slowing circulation in the pelvic area or causing congestion of the organs in the abdomen. As a result, the veins at the rectum swell and stretch to excess.

Local irritation and unrestrained eating and drinking: Cold or hot stimulation, constipation, diarrhea, excessive drinking, and eating too much pungent and spicy food are all likely to irritate the anus and rectum, causing the blood vessels to swell, affecting the reverse flow of blood in the veins and resulting in excessive stretching of the veins.

Manifestations and Symptoms

External hemorrhoids do not have obvious symptoms, but sufferers will experience a gritty or swollen feeling if they stand or walk for a long time.

Internal hemorrhoids do not cause any discomfort, but the main symptom is bleeding. With early-stage hemorrhoids, there may be a small amount of blood after bowel movements, or simply stools with blood streaks, blood accompanying stools, sprays or drips of bright red blood, or blood on the toilet paper.

Hand Reflexology and Acupressure

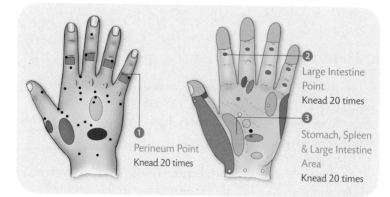

1 Perineum Point
Knead 20 times

2 Large Intestine Point
Knead 20 times

3 Stomach, Spleen & Large Intestine Area
Knead 20 times

Hand Exercises

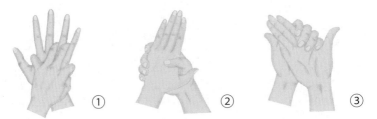

1. With your right palm facing down, lock the fingers of your left hand into those of the right hand; squeeze and press as much as you like.

2. With your right hand, hold onto your left hand horizontally; press the tips of the four fingers of the right hand onto the skin on the back of the left hand; in the meantime, press your left palm against your right palm as hard as you can.

3. Place the back of your right hand above your left palm, and bend the four fingers of your left hand to squeeze your right palm; in the meantime, press your right palm against your left hand.

Other Methods

For people affected with hemorrhoids, good dietary habits and a healthy lifestyle are important:

1. Eat more fresh vegetables and fruit rich in fibers and vitamins, and avoid spicy and irritating food.

2. Go to see a doctor and get appropriate treatment if you have persistent constipation; do not take laxatives or use enemas over an extended period of time, as doing so may desensitize the mucosa of the rectum, incapacitate the bowel, and worsen your constipation, eventually resulting in hemorrhoids.

Due to the high recurrence of hemorrhoids, measures should be taken to prevent them:

1. Take exercise, and increase the body's resistance to diseases.

2. Maintain a healthy lifestyle, such as avoiding alcohol and pungent and spicy food; eat more vegetables and fruit, and develop a fixed time for bowel movements.

Chapter Seven

Disorders of the Orthopedic and Genito-Urinary Systems

There are 206 bones in an adult human body. They are connected by joints and ligaments, all of which constitutes the skeleton and gives the human being its basic form. The skeletal system also protects the internal organs and supports the functions of athletic performance. The urinary system, consisting of the kidneys, ureter, bladder, and urinary tract, functions primarily for the purpose of excretion. The reproductive system, however, serves to continue the human race generation after generation through a variety of biological activities including insemination and conception. This chapter aims at improving the health of your orthopedic, urinary, and reproductive systems.

1. Cervical Spondylosis

Cervical spondylosis is a condition caused by stimulation and pressure on the roots of the nerves.

Chronic wear and tear is believed to be the primary cause of cervical spondylosis. It damages local ligaments, muscles, and joint capsules resulting in local edema and hemorrhage. Then, infection occurs and spurs may develop, affecting the local nerves and blood vessels. Acute and chronic neck injuries after prolonged periods of working with the head down, or incorrect posture, violent impact, cervical deterioration, trauma to the neck, and chronic soreness are all major causes of cervical spondylosis.

Manifestations and Symptoms

Its main symptoms are soreness of the head, neck, shoulders, back, and arms, with a stiff neck restricting movement; a heavy sensation in the shoulders and back; weak arms, numbness of the fingers, and an inability to grasp things firmly. The patient may sometimes experience vertigo and palpitations. If the condition is serious, the patient may experience light-headedness, headache, blurred vision, dry and swollen eyes that are hard to open, clogged ears, tinnitus, loss of balance, racing heart, nervousness, and bloating of the gastro-intestinal tract. Other symptoms include difficulty swallowing and voice loss. If long-term treatment is unsuccessful, the disease may trigger psychological symptoms such as insomnia, irritability, anger, anxiety, and depression.

Hand Reflexology and Acupressure

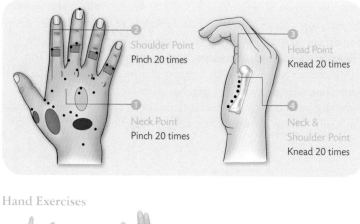

Shoulder Point
Pinch 20 times

Head Point
Knead 20 times

Neck Point
Pinch 20 times

Neck & Shoulder Point
Knead 20 times

Hand Exercises

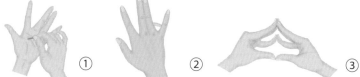

①   ②   ③

1. With your palm facing inward, spread out the fingers. Use a stick to jab the transverse creases of the thumb evenly from the top down.

2. With your palm facing outward, place a coin horizontally between the proximal phalanges of the little and ring fingers. Hold the coin there with force, and move it up to the fingertip.

3. Press your thumb and four fingers against each other to form an angle, and keep pressing to make it as large as you can through resistance.

Other Methods

1. During breaks at work, do some activities that help relax the cervical spine and prevent cervical spondylosis, such as folding the neck up and down, and turning your head to the left and right. Do this once or twice, and repeat it for 10 minutes every day.

2. Maintain a good sleeping posture. It is best to use a soft contoured pillow to keep the neck in its natural curve. The height of the pillow should be about 10 cm.

3. Maintain a good posture at work. Try to sit in a posture with your head neither tilting up nor lowering down. Move your neck after working for an hour, to give the ligaments and muscles a rest.

2. Frozen Shoulder

Frozen shoulder is a condition characterized by damage and wear and tear to the soft tissues, muscles, ligaments, tendons, synovial bursae, and joint capsules of the shoulders. This age-related deterioration gradually develops into a chronic non-bacterial inflammation around the shoulder's joint capsules and soft tissues.

Frozen shoulder is often found in people around 50 years of age. The causes are:

1. Prolonged periods of overwork and incorrect posture causing chronic strain injuries.

2. Injury to the upper limbs, meaning that the shoulder has to remain in a fixed position for a long period of time, causing the tissue around the shoulder to shrink and stick together.

3. Sudden injury to the shoulder due to strain, which is left untreated or treated incorrectly.

Manifestations and Symptoms

Shoulder pain is the most evident symptom. A pain begins somewhere in your shoulder, which is clearly related to an action or posture you have taken. As the condition progresses, the area of pain grows to involve the middle part of the upper arm, accompanied by limited movement of the shoulder. When the condition worsens, the affected arm cannot even move to brush the hair or wash the face.

Hand Reflexology and Acupressure

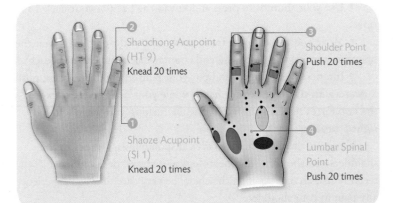

Shaochong Acupoint (HT 9)
Knead 20 times

Shoulder Point
Push 20 times

Shaoze Acupoint (SI 1)
Knead 20 times

Lumbar Spinal Point
Push 20 times

Hand Exercises

1. Bend the thumb and the fingers of your right hand slightly, forming a hollow fist, with the thumb and the little finger pinching each other.

2. With your right hand, hold onto your left hand horizontally, with the tips of the four fingers jabbing and pressing the skin of the left hand, while the left palm presses against the right hand.

3. Hold a stick with the tips of the index fingers and hold it there firmly. In the meantime, press the thumbs against each other.

Other Methods

Keep warm and avoid letting the shoulder catch cold. If you sit working at desk, or if your shoulders remain in the abduction position for a long time, adjust your posture from time to time to avoid chronic wear and tear and accumulative injuries.

Do exercises during work breaks to relax the shoulders and neck:

• Stand up straight; keep your hands down naturally, place your feet shoulder-width apart, and lean your head as far back as possible, while keeping your eyes fixed on one object for 15 seconds.

• Use your thumbs to press and knead the back of your neck 15 times.

• Move your head to the front, back, left, and right; then do it the opposite way; do this clockwise and counter-clockwise 10 times each.

• Interlock your fingers and put your palms behind the neck; push forward with the force of your hands while your neck goes backward, the two forces resisting each other, while turning your head left and right 5 times.

If you are diabetic, or have cervical spondylosis, injuries to the shoulders and the arms, and neurological diseases, or if you have recently had an operation on the chest, be very careful if you experience any pain in your shoulder.

3. Lumbar Disc Herniation

Lumbar disc herniation is a common illness that occurs when the inner nucleus pulposus ruptures from the annular tear and presses the nerve roots, causing a clinical syndrome characterized primarily by sciatica.

The deterioration of the lumbar disc usually starts when a person is in their 20s, compounded by accumulative injuries from daily life and work. When the disc is subject to repeated pressure, it buckles and twists, and the back of the annulus is likely to rupture. With repeated pressure, the rupture grows where the annulus becomes increasingly thinner. Any additional trauma can cause it to break, resulting in pain in the lower back radiating to the leg, or even causing neurological impairment.

Manifestations and Symptoms
Radiating pain that travels along the sciatic nerve, from the lower back and buttocks to the thigh, the leg, and the surface of the foot. The event of coughing, sneezing, bowel movements, and bending can exacerbate the pain. The pain increases when the patient is in motion, but will subside after rest. It occurs repeatedly.

Hand Reflexology and Acupressure

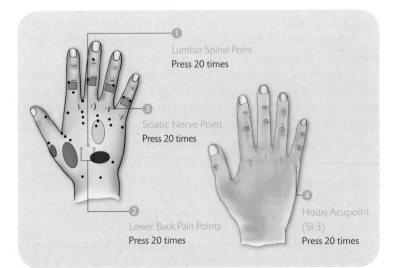

Lumbar Spinal Point
Press 20 times

Sciatic Nerve Point
Press 20 times

Lower Back Pain Points
Press 20 times

Houxi Acupoint
(SI 3)
Press 20 times

Hand Exercises

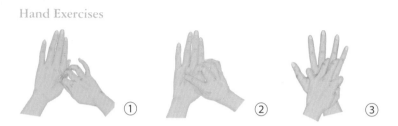

1. With your right thumb and index finger, pinch and pull the skin on the back of the left hand along the metacarpal bone of the index finger.

2. With your right thumb and index finger, pinch and pull the skin below the end of the proximal phalanx of the left ring finger.

3. With your right palm facing down, lock the fingers of your left hand into those of the right hand, and press and squeeze as you please.

Other Methods

1. Alternate work with rest; avoid staying in the same posture and repeating the same movement over an extended period of time.

2. People whose work requires bending at the waist or working at a desk for a prolonged period of time should adjust the height of their desk and chair to change posture. A 15-minute exercise session is recommended after 45 minutes of working sitting down.

3. People who have to bend very often should move regularly to stretch their back and open their chest, and should wear a wider belt.

4. Keep a healthy lifestyle; maintain regular meal times and bed times; avoid staying up late.

5. Exercise is a good way of prevention and cure, e.g., swimming and aerobics. Also, lie on your chest, lift up your head, arms, legs, and feet as high as you can; lift them up and put them down as one round, and do four groups of eight rounds each time, once or twice every day. This will help to prevent lumbar disc herniation.

4. Urinary Stones

Urinary stones indicate the presence of hard particles or deposits in the urinary system due to high urine concentration. The stones are found in the kidneys, ureter, and anywhere in the urinary tract.

Manifestations and Symptoms

Clinical manifestations may vary due to the different locations of the stones. Kidney stones and ureteral stones are typically characterized by renal colic and blood in the urine. At the onset, the patient will feel intense pain, either constant or intermittent, in the lower back, radiating along the ureter to places such as the iliac fossa, perineum, and scrotum. Before the onset, the patient usually has no symptoms, but suddenly experiences an intense bursting pain on one side of the lower back due to intense exercise, physical labor, or long-distance travel. It is often accompanied by fullness of the abdomen, nausea, vomiting, blood in the urine, pyuria, difficultly urinating, or interrupted urine flow.

Hand Reflexology and Acupressure

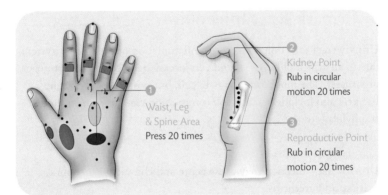

Waist, Leg & Spine Area
Press 20 times

Kidney Point
Rub in circular motion 20 times

Reproductive Point
Rub in circular motion 20 times

Hand Exercises

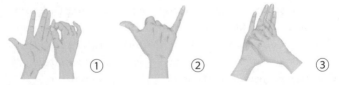

1. With your thumb and index finger, twist and press the little finger of the other hand in spiral rotation from the bottom up.

2. With your palm facing outwards, quickly contract the three fingers in the middle, making the Chinese finger-counting sign for "6." Do it six times.

3. With your right thumb and index finger, pinch the skin of the little finger along its metacarpus to the wrist crease.

Other Methods

In daily life, people with urinary stones should:

1. Lower their intake of animal protein, e.g., meat and offal.
2. Lower their intake of salt and maintain a light diet.
3. Drink light tea or water instead of strong tea.
4. Refrain from drinking milk less than 4 hours before sleep. The formation of kidney stones is due to a sudden increase of calcium in the urine. The peak time for calcium to exit the body is 2 to 3 hours after drinking milk. If you are sleeping at this time, the urine becomes concentrated and more calcium stays in the kidneys, increasing the likelihood that stones will form.

5. Urinary Tract Infection

Urinary tract infection refers to an inflammation of the urinary system due to an attack of bacteria (and very occasionally by fungus, protozoa, or viruses). The most common is E. coli, but possible contributing bacteria also include bacillus coli communior, bacillus proteus, and staphylococcus.

Manifestations and Symptoms

Urinary tract infection may cause acute and chronic pyelonephritis, cystitis, and urethritis.

Acute pyelonephritis: Systemic symptoms include sudden onset, chills, shaking, feverish sensation, discomfort across the body, headache, fatigue, poor appetite, nausea, vomiting, lower back pain, and discomfort in the kidney area. Symptoms in the urinary system include bladder inflammation leading to urinary urgency, frequent or painful urination, lower back pain, and/or lower abdominal pain.

Chronic pyelonephritis: Manifestations may be similar to acute pyelonephritis but much less severe, with no fever, systemic discomfort, or headache. Signs of urinary tract infection: Only a small number of patients have intermittent symptoms of pyelonephritis, but more common is the presence of intermittent symptomless bacteria in the urine and/or intermittent urine urgency, frequent urination, discomfort in the lower back, and/or intermittent low-grade fever. Chronic interstitial nephritis-related manifestations are hypertension, frequent urination, increased urination at night, higher occurrence of dehydration. Chronic kidney disease-related signs are a puffy face in the morning, frequent urination at night, and back pain.

Cystitis and urethritis: Manifestations are primarily frequent, urgent, and painful urination, as well as pain in the bladder area.

Hand Reflexology and Acupressure

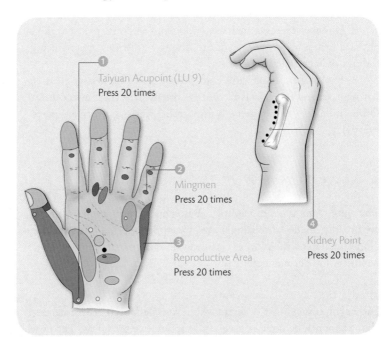

① Taiyuan Acupoint (LU 9)
Press 20 times

② Mingmen
Press 20 times

③ Reproductive Area
Press 20 times

④ Kidney Point
Press 20 times

Hand Exercises

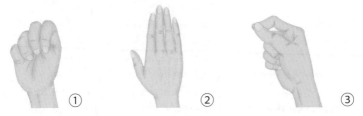

① ② ③

1. Make a fist with the palm faces inward. Withdraw the thumb to tuck it between the ring finger and the little finger, and contract and

squeeze the remaining four fingers with force.

2. Place a coin vertically between the proximal phalanges of the little finger and the index finger.

3. Bend the five digits of your right hand slightly, forming a hollow fist, and align your thumb and index finger to make the tips jab each other.

Other Methods

1. Avoid negative emotions and keep a positive outlook.

2. Do more exercise, such as jogging and walking, to strength your physical fitness and improve your resistance to disease, thus reducing the risk of bacterial infection.

3. For women, make sure your private parts are always clean. For men, a long foreskin is likely to cause urinary tract infections, so maintaining good hygiene is important; wash your private parts every day.

6. Nephritis

There are many types of nephritis. Based on the initial causes, they are broadly divided into congenital glomerulonephritis and secondary glomerulonephritis. Another classification is based on duration: acute nephritis and chronic nephritis.

Manifestations and Symptoms

Early symptoms: Most sufferers will have experienced other infection about a month before its onset, e.g., suppurative tonsillitis. The onset can be sudden, accompanied by high fever. It can also be gradual and can go unnoticed.

Hypertension: One of the most typical signs of nephritis.

Swelling: About half of those affected experience swelling when urination decreases. The swelling is more evident in the face and the lower extremities, and is difficult to alleviate once it has begun.

Symptoms in the neurological system: The primary signs are headache, nausea, vomiting, insomnia, and decreased thinking ability. In serious cases, the sufferer may experience visual impairment, or even amaurosis, fainting, and seizures.

Anemia: Sufferers of nephritis are often found to have anemia, and may experience fatigue and dizziness.

Hand Reflexology and Acupressure

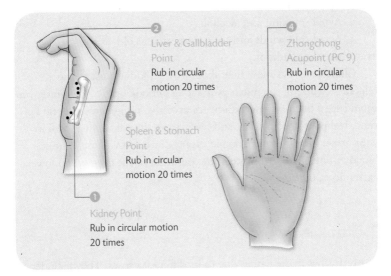

Hand Exercises

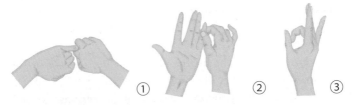

1. Use the five digits of your right hand to pull away the proximal phalanx of the left little finger slowly 15 times.

2. With your thumb and index finger, hold the proximal phalanx of the little finger of the other hand, and twist and pull it in a spiral rotation.

3. Open your palm and abruptly retract your middle finger toward the thumb while keeping the index, ring, and little fingers straight.

Other Methods

Patients should regulate their life schedule and cultivate a healthy lifestyle:

1. Keep a regular schedule and maintain a healthy lifestyle; do not overwork, as excessive fatigue is likely to worsen the condition.

2. Do aerobics and exercises for physical fitness.

3. Maintain a pleasant mood.

4. Avoid smoking and alcohol.

5. Avoid cold winds and try not to catch a cold, as this can exacerbate the condition.

Clinical surveys show that about 70% of kidney disease cases are related to working too much over a long period of time. Therefore, you should see a doctor if you experience excessive fatigue over a period of time, feel pain in your waist and back, experience increased foam in your urine, increased urination at night, decreased volume of urine, bloody urine, increased proteinuria, puffiness of the eyelids and lower extremities, or dizziness.

7. Prostatitis

Prostatitis has many names due to its different causes. They include non-specific bacterial prostatitis, idiopathic bacterial prostatitis, specific prostatitis, non-specific granulomatous prostatitis, prostate by other pathogens, and prostate congestion.

Manifestations and Symptoms

Often accompanied by urgent and frequent urination, and pain in the private parts when urinating. The condition may manifest as chills and high fever, accompanied by constant and evident lower urinary tract infection, dribbling urination, cloudy urine, and inflamed discharge from the urinary tract, as well as lethargy and fatigue, and aversion to cold in the lower back and knees. Illnesses such as acute cystitis may occur at the same time.

Acute inflammation may turn chronic either because the condition becomes more serious or before the treatment can run its course and cure the problem. In the case of acute prostatitis turning chronic, the primary signs are pain in the pelvis and abnormal urination. Chronic pain lasts for an extended period of time and cannot be healed. The affected may experience declining quality of life, and further problems such as sexual dysfunction, anxiety, depression, insomnia, and memory problems.

Hand Reflexology and Acupressure

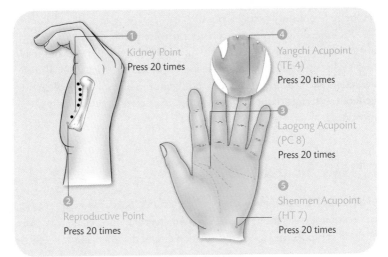

Kidney Point
Press 20 times

Yangchi Acupoint
(TE 4)
Press 20 times

Laogong Acupoint
(PC 8)
Press 20 times

Reproductive Point
Press 20 times

Shenmen Acupoint
(HT 7)
Press 20 times

Hand Exercises

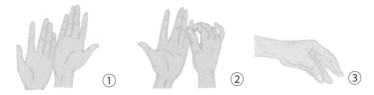

1. With your palms facing up and the heels of the palms pressing against each other, rub them back and forth as many times as you want.

2. With your thumb and index finger, hold the proximal phalanx of the little finger of the other hand, and press and twist it in a spiral rotation.

3. Bend the fingers of your left hand slightly, forming a hollow fist, then pinch the tips of your thumb and little finger together.

Other Methods

If you experience urgent and frequent urination, you should see a doctor as soon as you can during the acute onset. Void your bowels regularly, drink more water, and urinate more often.

Pay attention to the following in your daily life to avoid triggering prostatitis: Excessive sexual activity, forced termination of sexual intercourse, excessive masturbation, an over-restrained sex life, and prolonged voluntary sexual arousal.

Prolonged direct pressure on your private parts, such as cycling, horse riding, and sitting, are likely to cause repeated damage and may lead to a congested prostate, resulting in prostatitis. Also, unhealthy life habits such as alcoholism and indulgence in oily food will likely generate systemic damp-heat in your reproductive organs, causing prostatitis.

8. Male Sexual Dysfunction

Male sexual function includes five components: Sexual arousal, getting an erection, penetration, maintaining an erection, and ejaculation. Any of these components can be dysfunctional, and disorders are collectively known as male sexual dysfunction.

Manifestations and Symptoms

Common dysfunctions include low libido, sexual aversion, hyper-arousal and sexual desire disorders, and dysfunctional erection, penetration, and ejaculation. Ejaculation dysfunction includes premature ejaculation, inhibited ejaculation, and retrograde ejaculation.

Hand Reflexology and Acupressure

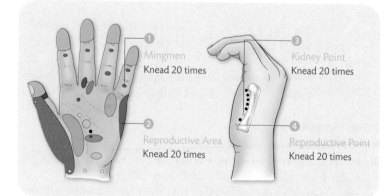

1 Mingmen
Knead 20 times

2 Reproductive Area
Knead 20 times

3 Kidney Point
Knead 20 times

4 Reproductive Point
Knead 20 times

Hand Exercises

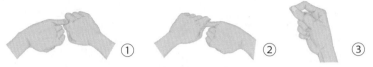

1. With the five digits of your right hand, pull the proximal phalanx of the left little finger slowly 15 times.

2. With the five digits of your left hand, pull the proximal phalanx of the right little finger slowly 15 times.

3. Bend the digits of your right hand slightly, forming a hollow fist. Press the thumb and the index finger against each other so that the tips pinch each other.

Other Methods

Maintain emotional balance. When stressed, stay calm and think rationally. Learn to relax and adjust tension at all times, and avoid anxious or depressive moods.

Steer clear of unhealthy lifestyles and diets. Avoid unnecessary socializing and alcoholism, and control your food intake; understand dangers of smoking, and make a concerted effort to quit. Be focused while having intercourse; sleep in separate beds for a while to avoid too much sexual stimulation and allow your nervous system and sex organs to rest. Research shows that these measures are an effective way of preventing and treating sexual dysfunction. Eat more food that tonifies *yang*, such as lamb, sparrow, and walnuts, as well as food that contains arginine, e.g., Chinese yam, ginkgo seeds, frozen tofu, eel, sea cucumber, squid, and octopus.

Chapter Eight

Gynecological Diseases and Disorders

Problems with the female reproductive system are known as gynecological diseases and disorders. They are common, and often cause great discomfort to women. Due to limited knowledge of such matters, many women do not have adequate resources to take care of their bodies. Unhealthy lifestyles make things even worse. Many women are riddled with illnesses of various kinds, and suffer the consequences of long and ineffective treatments, resulting in inconveniences in their life and work. This chapter aims to improve women's health through the practice of hand reflexology and acupressure.

1. Mammary Gland Hyperplasia

Mammary gland hyperplasia is a pathological process in which the glandular tissues and the middle and end parts of the lactiferous ducts expand, grow too much, and experience cystic change.

Modern medical science holds that one of the primary causes of mammary gland hyperplasia are infertility among older women, irregular sexual intercourse, termination of pregnancy, and unhealthy lifestyles such as excessive intake of high-fat and high-calorie food, alcoholism, and smoking. Other factors include external living environments and genetic inheritance.

Manifestations and Symptoms

Lumps in the breast: Tough, cyst-like nodules of various sizes, which move around and are not attached to the skin or the tissues deeper in the breast. The lumps may grow on one side or both sides, and can be single or multiple. They usually appear in the outer, upper quadrant of the breast. These lumps change form with the menstrual cycle: They are bigger and tougher prior to menstruation, and smaller and softer afterwards.

Armpits: The patient usually experiences sore and swelling sensations, but the lymph nodes in the armpit do not swell or grow.

Nipple discharge: Occasional nipple discharge of yellow or greenish yellow fluid, or colorless serous effusion. If the discharge turns reddish or brownish, you should see a doctor.

Hand Reflexology and Acupressure

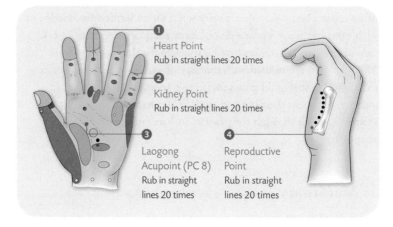

Heart Point
Rub in straight lines 20 times

Kidney Point
Rub in straight lines 20 times

Laogong Acupoint (PC 8)
Rub in straight lines 20 times

Reproductive Point
Rub in straight lines 20 times

Hand Exercises

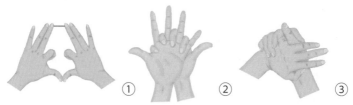

1. Hold a stick between the tips of both middle fingers. Press the thumbs of both hands against each other, with both index fingers withdrawn.

2. With your left palm up, spread out the five digits. Interlock the fingers of your right hand with those of the left hand from behind, pressing and jabbing the left hand with force.

3. With your right palm, hold onto your left palm horizontally and press the withdrawn left little finger underneath the right palm; attach the other three fingers of your left hand to the back of your right hand and press it.

Other Methods

Women suffering from mammary gland hyperplasia should be vigilant in all of the following situations: A long history of mammary gland hyperplasia; overgrowth of nodules (which are many and evident) if touched; aged between 40 and 60 (an age bracket with a high incidence of cancer); a family history of breast cancer.

Special attention should be paid to painless lumps. Breast cancer lumps may not be painful in the early stage. However, once you feel pain, the cancer may have entered the middle or later stages. Go to a specialized hospital for examination to rule out the possibility of cancer.

2. Abnormal Menstruation

Abnormal menstruation refers to longer or shorter menstrual cycles than usual, heavier or lighter menstrual flow than usual, or changes in the nature of the discharge, sometime accompanied by discomfort.

It is caused by the following:

• Neuroendocrine dysfunction: Unstable function or deficiency of the posterior pituitary-ovarian axis results in abnormal periods.

• Long-term depression, anger, or severe emotional and psychological trauma could also cause abnormal menstruation or period cramps and amenorrhea.

• Organic diseases: Local inflammation of the reproductive organs, tumors and abnormal development, malnutrition, disorders of the brain, liver and blood diseases.

Manifestations and Symptoms
The condition is characterized by disorders in menstruation cycles and the volume of blood discharge:

1. Irregular uterine bleeding: Excess period discharge or extremely long periods, often found with uterine fibroids, endometrial polyps, and endometriosis.

2. Functional uterine bleeding: Disorders of the endocrine system, but no signs of physical diseases of the reproductive organs.

3. Vaginal bleeding after menopause: This refers to bleeding six months after menstruation has ceased. It is often caused by malignant tumor or inflammation.

4. Amenorrhea: Females over 18 years of age who have never had periods are considered as having congenital amenorrhea; menstruation stops any time after the first period and before menopause (excluding pregnancy or breastfeeding), with a duration of six months or longer; these people are considered to have secondary amenorrhea.

Hand Reflexology and Acupressure

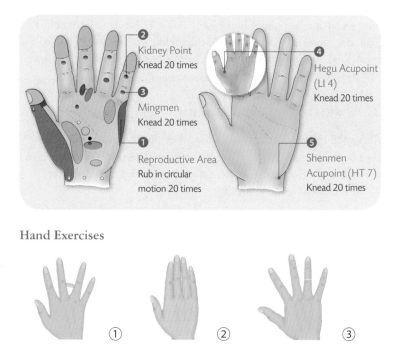

Kidney Point
Knead 20 times

Mingmen
Knead 20 times

Reproductive Area
Rub in circular
motion 20 times

Hegu Acupoint
(LI 4)
Knead 20 times

Shenmen
Acupoint (HT 7)
Knead 20 times

Hand Exercises

① ② ③

1. With your palm facing outward, place a coin horizontally between the proximal phalanges of your middle and ring fingers. Keep it there firmly, and then move it upward.

2. With your palm facing outward, place a coin between the proximal phalanges of the ring and little fingers. Keep it there firmly, and then move it up and down without it falling off.

3. Put a ring on the middle phalanx of the ring finger, and use your middle or little finger to turn it, stimulating the finger.

Other Methods

Sufferers of abnormal menstruation should do the following:

1. Keep warm, and prevent cold from getting into the body.

2. Pay attention to your diet and avoid raw and cold food, as coldness tends to congeal the blood and thus exacerbate period cramps.

3. Take more rest and avoid fatigue.

4. Keep your emotions in check and avoid violent mood swings. Maintain a good mood.

3. Uterine Fibroids

Uterine fibroids are among the most common benign tumors of the female reproductive organs, consisting of lumps that grow in the uterus due to smooth muscle cell proliferation.

Many clinical observations and experiments show that the growth of uterine fibroids depends on female hormones. Patients often have ovarian hyperemia, swelling of the ovaries, and an excess of endometrial hyperplasia. All these signs indicate an abnormally high level of female hormones.

Manifestations and Symptoms

Uterine fibroids typically manifest as:

1. Excessively heavy periods and secondary anemia; prolonged duration of periods, and shorter intervals between periods; irregular or non-stop flow of blood.

2. Lumps in the lower abdomen, and increased leucorrhea discharge.

3. Fibroids in the front wall of the uterine may suppress the bladder, causing a more frequent and urgent need to urinate.

4. They may also cause conditions such as difficult urination, urinary retention, a heavy and distended lower abdomen, and constipation. In severe cases, infertility and miscarriage are likely.

Some people ignore the existence of uterine fibroids, believing that they are benign tumors. However, they may trigger gynecological infections such as adnexitis and pelvic inflammatory disease. Uterine fibroids can have complications primarily caused by torsion of the pedicle in ovarian tumors, or acute endometritis.

Hand Reflexology and Acupressure

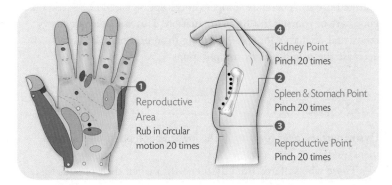

❶ Reproductive Area
Rub in circular motion 20 times

❷ Spleen & Stomach Point
Pinch 20 times

❸ Reproductive Point
Pinch 20 times

❹ Kidney Point
Pinch 20 times

Hand Exercises

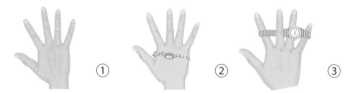

1. Put a ring on the middle phalanx of the ring finger, and turn it with your hand to stimulate the finger.

2. Put a wristwatch or an elastic band on your palm, and stretch and contract your hand.

3. Put a wristwatch or an elastic band on the index, ring, and little fingers, leaving the middle finger above the strap. Stretch your fingers as far as you can.

Other Methods

Special care should be given to your daily diet:

1. Eat light food with low salt and oil; avoid lamb, shrimps, prawns, crab, eel, salted fish, and snakehead fish, as they can trigger certain diseases and conditions.

2. Avoid irritating food and drinks such as chili pepper, Sichuan pepper, raw scallions, and liquor.

3. Avoid food such as longan, dates, gelatine from donkey skin, and royal jelly, as they contain heat and hormones, and cause congealing.

In addition, have regular checkups and seek appropriate treatment based on the progression of the disease. Terminating a pregnancy may damage the uterus and cervix, and thus increase the risk of uterine fibroids. Therefore, proper contraception should be used. Take good care of yourself during menstruation. This will alleviate heavy menstrual discharge for those suffering from uterine polyps, and decrease the risk of serious complications.

4. Dysmenorrhea

Dysmenorrhea refer to pains in the lower abdomen in the course of menstruation.

Those who suffered from dysmenorrhea when their periods first started but whose reproductive organs show no signs of organic disease are considered to have congenital dysmenorrhea. When dysmenorrhea occurs because of physiological pathogens in the reproductive organs, this is called secondary dysmenorrhea. Reproductive diseases include uterine hypoplasia, cervical stenosis, and endometriosis. Dysmenorrhea may also result from mental or physiological factors, such as excessive stress, nervousness, chronic diseases, and anemia.

Manifestations and Symptoms

In the first two days of menstruation, the patient may feel throbbing or cramping pain in the lower abdomen. The pain may radiate to the patient's vulva, anus, and lower back, and is usually accompanied by nausea, vomiting, headache, dizziness, pale complexion, sweating, and cold hands and feet. The pain will disappear when the period ends.

Dysmenorrhea is only one of many signs of gynecological diseases, and may conceal the existence of other issues. Seek proper medical treatment, and don't allow your condition to deteriorate. In general, fever during menstruation accompanied by cramping pain in the lower abdomen usually suggests that you have pelvic inflammatory disease. If your menstrual blood is light brown, or has an abnormal odor, accompanied by rising temperature and lower abdominal pain, it is likely that you have endometritis. Likewise, if your period pains grow longer and more severe, you may have endometriosis.

Hand Reflexology and Acupressure

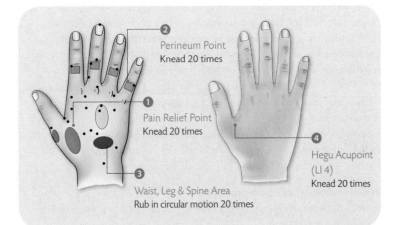

❷ Perineum Point
Knead 20 times

❶ Pain Relief Point
Knead 20 times

❹ Hegu Acupoint
(LI 4)
Knead 20 times

❸ Waist, Leg & Spine Area
Rub in circular motion 20 times

Hand Exercises

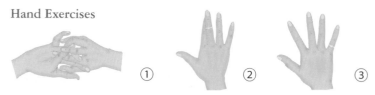

1. Attach both thumbs and little fingers to each other, and lock the remaining fingers into one another.

2. Put a ring on the middle phalanx of your middle finger, and use the other hand to move it up and down.

3. Put the ring on the proximal phalanx of your little finger and move it up and down.

Other Methods
Exercises can help restore the uterus to its normal position:

1. Lie on your back with your legs together. Raise your knees slightly, and keep them there while doing diaphragmatic breathing 20 times. Do this two to three times daily. Diaphragmatic breathing is a style of deep breathing in which inhalation does not expand the chest but raises the abdomen, and exhalation contracts the abdomen instead of the chest.

2. Stand up straight, lift up your heels, and then drop them down. Repeat this 20 times. Do this exercise three times every day.

5. Female Infertility

If a woman is not able to get pregnant after more than two years of unprotected sex with her spouse (who has normal reproductive function), this is considered to be primary infertility. If a woman cannot conceive more than two years after giving birth, abortion, or miscarriage, this is called secondary infertility.

Many factors can cause female infertility. They include conditions such as congenital absence of ovaries, polycystic ovaries, salpingitis, endometriosis, uterine fibroids, cervical inflammation, and cervical stenosis. Psychological factors may also affect a woman's chances of getting pregnant. Therefore, it is of critical importance that you remain psychologically and emotionally healthy.

Manifestations and Symptoms
A healthy woman trying to conceive for more than two years is not able to get pregnant.

Hand Reflexology and Acupressure

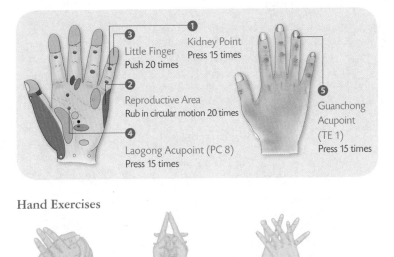

❸ Little Finger
Push 20 times

❶ Kidney Point
Press 15 times

❷ Reproductive Area
Rub in circular motion 20 times

❹ Laogong Acupoint (PC 8)
Press 15 times

❺ Guanchong Acupoint (TE 1)
Press 15 times

Hand Exercises

① ② ③

1. With your right palm up, bend the little finger inward. With your left hand, cover the right palm from above, pressing the little finger of the right hand.

2. With your palms facing each other, bend both thumbs and index fingers. Interlock the ring fingers and little fingers, and the fingertips of both hands press or squeeze the points they touch with force.

3. With your left palm down, spread out the five digits. With your right hand, press the left palm, and spread out the five digits and rub the left hand in a circular motion 20 times.

Other Methods

1. Increase dietary nutrition by taking multivitamins such as Vitamins A, B, C, and E, to prepare your body for pregnancy.

2. Avoid unhealthy environments, and take preventative measures when you are in a profession that may have adverse effects on pregnancy.

3. The female reproductive tract is susceptible to infection and blocked fallopian tubes after curettage. Curettage is also likely to damage the uterus and kidneys, leading to endocrine disorders and thus affecting your chances of pregnancy. Lack of rest after curettage can make it harder to get pregnant.

4. Women with infertility issues may also suffer from emotional distress, and should be treated with love and care.

Chapter Nine

Skin Conditions and Diseases of the Nose, Eyes, Throat, and Teeth

The skin is the largest organ in the human body. It prevents the internal organs and tissues from being attacked physically, mechanically, chemically, and by pathogenic microorganisms. The skin functions as a barrier to the outside world in two ways: It prevents the loss of bodily fluids, electrolytes, and other substances, and stops the invasion of external harmful substances. It retains the internal stability of the body, provides biological protection, and participates in the metabolic process. The health of the skin and the facial organs is not only crucial to the overall health of a human being, but is also related to the aesthetics of external appearance. By understanding the hand reflexology and acupressure in this chapter, you will learn how to improve the health of your skin and your facial organs, for internal and external vibrancy.

1. Eczema

Eczema is one of the most common inflammatory skin diseases, and can either be acute or chronic.

The causes of eczema can be internal and external.

External triggers: Chemical irritants such as dyes, medicine, paint, soap, detergent, cosmetics; sunlight, UV rays, extremely low temperatures, extreme heat, dryness and humidity, and physical irritants such as animal hair, feathers, and glass fibers.

Internal triggers: Chronic diseases such as gastrointestinal disorders, intestinal parasites, chronic alcohol intoxication, metabolic dysfunction, and endocrine disorders, and emotional problems such as nervousness, insomnia, and fatigue.

Manifestations and Symptoms
Primary manifestations include intense itching, and multiple forms of skin lesions that are symmetrical in distribution with a tendency to ooze. The course of the disease is long, and it can reoccur from time to time.

Acute Eczema: Skin patches with red papule; papule with pus-filled blisters, with clear dots or small patches of erosion that weep fluid and form scabs. Acute eczema results in skin lesions of multiple forms, and can recur, which may lead to chronic eczema.

Chronic Eczema: Inefficient treatment and repeated recurrence of acute and sub-acute eczema can result in chronic eczema. Skin lesions turn dark red, brownish red, or maculopapular. The patches often merge and thicken, becoming moss-like with scales, scratches, and blood crust on the skin surface. It is usually dotted with papules and sporadic maculopapulae. Itching can sometimes be unbearable, and the condition often worsens after taking a bath, drinking alcohol, overheating in bed, and emotional stress. It can sometimes affect a patient's sleep. Patches of chronic eczema are self-limiting, with clear edges. They are moist, and thicken over time.

Hand Reflexology and Acupressure

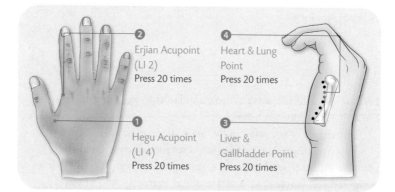

2 Erjian Acupoint (LI 2) Press 20 times

4 Heart & Lung Point Press 20 times

1 Hegu Acupoint (LI 4) Press 20 times

3 Liver & Gallbladder Point Press 20 times

Hand Exercises

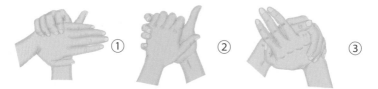

① ② ③

1. With your right hand, clasp the left palm positioned horizontally. With the four fingers of the right hand, clasp the back of the left palm, jabbing and pressing.

2. With your right palm, clasp the left palm horizontally. With the five digits of both hands, press the back of the other palm with force.

3. With your right palm up, withdraw the little finger; your left hand covers the right palm from above. Press the back of the right hand and squeeze the withdrawn little finger.

Other Methods

Avoid local irritation such as scratching, soap, hot baths, wiping with force, and inappropriate treatment. Avoid spicy and irritating food and alcohol. In the course of an acute outbreak, do not undergo immunization; an infant should not be vaccinated if suffering from eczema.

For young children suffering from eczema, the following measures are recommended:

1. Avoid using overheated water for baths, and do not use soap.
2. Avoid excessive exposure to the sun.
3. Avoid direct contact with clothes made from coarse cotton or synthetic fabrics, otherwise the condition could worsen.
4. Take sedative medicine as prescribed by the doctor before going to bed, as itching will affect sleep.
5. Trim children's fingernails, and wrap their fingers with gauze so they don't scratch themselves.
6. Avoid the chickenpox vaccine until the eczema has healed.

2. Urticaria

Urticaria is a common skin allergy. Clinically, it is divided into common urticaria, cold urticaria, and sunlight urticaria.

Many things can trigger this dermatologic condition: food such as fish, shrimps/prawns, crab, and eggs; allergies, self-immune problems, allergens in the air, infection, physical irritation, bug bites, and even some spicy condiments. Medicines such as penicillin and sulphanilamide may also trigger urticaria via the patient's immune system. Infections by viruses, bacteria, fungus, and parasites may also cause it.

Manifestations and Symptoms

The clinical manifestation of the disease is the sudden appearance of patches or groups of skin wheals that are unusually itchy, accompanied by fever, swollen joints, headache, nausea, vomiting, abdominal pain, diarrhea, and palpitations.

Wheals are of different shapes and sizes. They can be bright red or pale, and may disappear on their own. An individual wheal will not exist for more than 36 hours. No traces are left when they subside. If urticaria occurs in the throat, it may cause breathing trouble; if it is in the stomach and intestines, it may cause nausea, vomiting, and abdominal pain.

Hand Reflexology and Acupressure

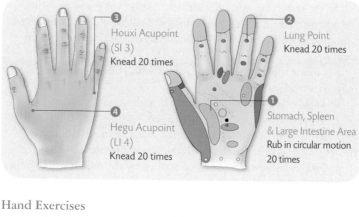

Houxi Acupoint
(SI 3)
Knead 20 times

Lung Point
Knead 20 times

Hegu Acupoint
(LI 4)
Knead 20 times

Stomach, Spleen
& Large Intestine Area
Rub in circular motion
20 times

Hand Exercises

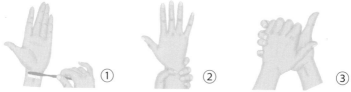

1. Brush your wrist crease with a toothbrush to the left and right, 30 times.

2. Stretch your right palm out, facing against you. Your left hand holds the right wrist horizontally to keep it in place, and then turn your right palm clockwise and counter-clockwise 10 times each.

3. Your right palm clasps the left palm horizontally. With the five digits of both hands, tightly clasp the back of the other palm, and press hard.

Other Methods

Patients with urticaria should avoid scratching the affected area. Do not apply warm compression in the affected area either. Follow a diet with few or no artificial additives. Eat fresh vegetables and fruit, including grapes, seaweed, tomatoes, sesame, cucumbers, carrots, bananas, and green beans. Wear a mask when going out to prevent other infections.

The following measures can be taken to prevent recurrence after the disease is cured:

1. Keep a fixed bedtime and time to get up. In spring and summer, go to bed late and get up early; in the fall, go to bed early and get up early; in winter, go to bed early but get up late.

2. Avoid keeping pets such as cats and dogs at home. Keep the house and carpets clean. Those who have a history of allergies should stay away from flowers and plants to avoid being affected by pollen.

3. For those whose urticaria may be triggered by contact, try to avoid soap containing perfumes, and avoid contact with chemical materials such as rubber and dye.

3. Acne

Acne, also known as acne vulgaris, is a chronic skin condition caused by sebaceous follicles. It usually occurs on the face, chest, and back, characterized by pimples, bumps, papules, nodules, and cystic lesions. It happens most commonly among young people.

There are many causes of acne. Traditional Chinese Medicine holds that it happens when the heat-wind passing the lung meridian is blocked by the skin. Pathogens include the patient's hormone levels, excessive sebum secretion, proliferation of propionibacterium acne, and inflammation and abnormal keratoses of the pilosebaceous ducts. Sometimes, excessive intake of rich, oily, and spicy food results in the rise of damp-heat in the body, causing an outbreak on the face. In addition, characterized by the rising *yang*-heat in the body, young blood fights wind-cold; however, when *yang*-heat is blocked in the skin, acne can occur.

Manifestations and Symptoms

First, a skin lesion appears, either whiteheads or blackheads. They are neither red nor raised above the skin, and too few in numbers to be visible. Open plugged pores have tips of a yellowish white color, but can turn black due to pigmentation. The spot has a black head, but when squeezed, its end appears as a semi-transparent white fat bolt. Pimples are the initial damage to the skin before they turn into acne. When the situation deteriorates, they become inflamed papules, and appear as red papules, pustules, nodules, abscesses, cysts, and scar.

Skin lesions often happen on the face, particularly on the forehead, cheeks, and chin. They also occur on the chest, back, and shoulders where sebum glands are numerous. Skin lesions usually appear symmetrically. Occasionally they also grow on other parts of the body. Acne lesions have no symptoms, but the patient may feel pain when the infection becomes more evident.

Hand Reflexology and Acupressure

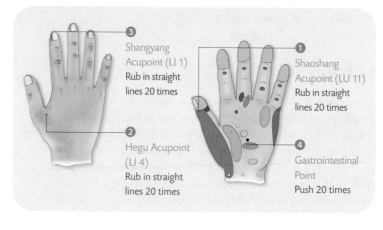

Shangyang Acupoint (LI 1)
Rub in straight lines 20 times

Shaoshang Acupoint (LU 11)
Rub in straight lines 20 times

Hegu Acupoint (LI 4)
Rub in straight lines 20 times

Gastrointestinal Point
Push 20 times

Hand Exercises

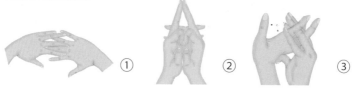

1. With your palms facing down, spread the fingers out. Interlock them, and press them against one another with force.

2. With your palms facing each other, bend both thumbs and index fingers; with the middle fingers facing each other, interlock the ring finger and the little fingers; press the tips of the middle fingers hard against each other.

3. With your right palm facing up, lock your left hand into the right hand from behind; with both hands, use the force of the fingers to press against each other; the right palm pulls forward and the left pulls back.

Other Methods

1. Try not to stay up late. Make sure you have plenty of sleep. Unhealthy lifestyles and late nights will exacerbate acne.

2. Maintain a cheerful mood, and avoid anxiety and mood swings.

3. Wash your face twice or three times a day with mild soap and warm water. There is no need for special soap during treatment, but when the condition becomes severe, use a medicinal liquid prescribed by your doctor to wash the affected area.

4. If the affected has oily skin, more care should be taken, because active secretion of sebum demands that the skin be left untouched; massage will only encourage the secretion of sebum.

5. Wash your hair frequently. Do not have bangs, and do not let your hair touch your face. This will cause a build-up of acne-causing grease.

6. Do not use foundation or cosmetics to cover facial acne. It will only block the pores and worsen the condition.

4. Psoriasis

Psoriasis is a skin condition characterized by patches of red skin and shining silvery scales.

Its primary causes are as follows:

1. Genetics: Those with a family history of psoriasis have a greater risk of being affected.

2. People who have suffered from tonsillitis, otitis media, and colds are also at higher risk of developing psoriasis.

3. Sometimes infections in the gastrointestinal, respiratory, sinus and genito-urinary systems may exacerbate psoriasis.

4. Emotional stress, anxiety, depression, and fear can also trigger or exacerbate psoriasis. The disease will worsen a few weeks or months after an episode of emotional stress.

Manifestations and Symptoms

Psoriasis often appears on the scalp, torso, and backside of the limbs as red patches that gradually grow and merge into scaly patches or plaques with clear borders. At the base of the affected area, there is moist skin. On the surface of the skin are thick, irregular silvery scales. When removing a scale you will see a red membrane, and when removing the membrane you will see petechiae. Features of this disease are white scales, shiny membranes, and punctuated red spots.

Hand Reflexology and Acupressure

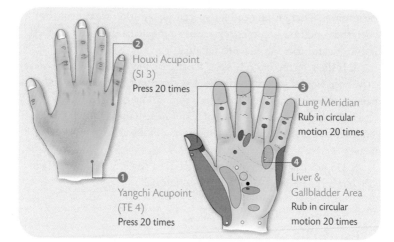

❷ Houxi Acupoint (SI 3)
Press 20 times

❸ Lung Meridian
Rub in circular motion 20 times

❶ Yangchi Acupoint (TE 4)
Press 20 times

❹ Liver & Gallbladder Area
Rub in circular motion 20 times

Hand Exercises

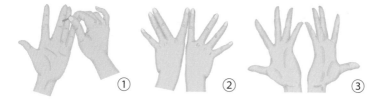

① ② ③

1. Use a stick to jab the middle finger evenly, from the fingertip downward.

2. With your palms facing down, withdraw both thumbs and align both hands side by side. Stretch out the remaining four fingers abruptly. The motion should have a strong impact.

3. With your palms facing up, spread the fingers and stretch both thumbs outward. Align the ulnar sides of the hands as an axis, and turn the palms downward as much as you can.

Other Methods

1. Prevent infection. Local infection, particularly tonsillitis, is a major

trigger of psoriasis. It is crucial that wounds and inflammation be cleaned promptly in the case of suppurative tonsillitis and similar illnesses.

2. Learn to adjust your emotions and stay optimistic; remain peaceful and calm.

3. Take enough rest and do adequate exercise to strengthen your physical fitness against diseases.

4. Keep healthy dietary habits. Try not to consume alcohol and smoke; avoid spicy and irritating food, and do not eat seafood and lamb.

5. Regularly take folic acid, and Vitamins A, C, and B$_{12}$.

5. Tonsillitis

Modern medical science holds that tonsillitis is the result of delayed treatment of acute tonsillitis, which is a non-specific acute inflammation of the palatine tonsils that is often found in children and adolescents but is rare among people who are 50 and above.

With excessive fatigue, smoking or alcohol, or cold and damp conditions, the body may lose its resistance to diseases, and the tonsil is thus likely to be affected by bacteria and inflammations.

Sometimes, after the onset of infectious diseases such as scarlet fever, diphtheria, measles, and flu, the condition may gradually become chronic. Bacteria such as staphylococcus and streptococcus pneumoniae may also trigger tonsillitis. Among them, the most common is Group A hemolytic streptococci.

Manifestations and Symptoms

Acute onset, severe chills, and high fever with the temperature reaching 39 to 40 ℃ . With young children, their temperature could be so high as to cause seizures, vomiting, coma, poor appetite, constipation, and systemic soreness and feebleness; evident pain in the throat, particularly when swallowing. When severe, the pain may radiate to the ear. Young children may cry and scream when trying to swallow. Children may suffer sleep disruption, because swollen tonsils block their airways.

Hand Reflexology and Acupressure

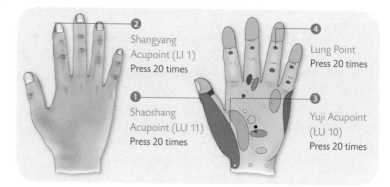

Shangyang
Acupoint (LI 1)
Press 20 times

Lung Point
Press 20 times

Shaoshang
Acupoint (LU 11)
Press 20 times

Yuji Acupoint
(LU 10)
Press 20 times

Hand Exercises

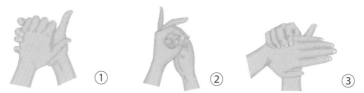

1. Your right palm holds onto your left palm horizontally; the five digits clasp the back of the other palm tightly and press hard.

2. Bring the five digits of your right hand together and wrap them with your left palm; repeatedly squeeze them and then release.

3. With your right hand, clasp your left palm positioned horizontally; with the four right fingers, clasp the back of the left palm, and jab and press down.

Other Methods

Do more exercise to strengthen your physical fitness and improve the body's resistance to diseases. Wear more clothes when temperatures are low. As chronic tonsillitis is contagious and may trigger chronic infections in the ear, nose, and throat, as well as arthritis, nephritis, and rheumatic heart disease, a tonsillectomy may be necessary.

6. Allergic Rhinitis

Allergic rhinitis is a hypersensitive reaction to certain allergens by people with particular constitutions, often the young.

It is mainly caused by pollen as the seasons change, e.g., from trees, wild grass, and agricultural crops. Perennial allergic rhinitis, however, is related to the perennial allergens in daily life, such as dust and dust mites in the house, fungi, animal hair and dander, feathers, and cotton fibers. Meanwhile, patients with atopic constitutions are usually found to have a family history of such allergies.

Manifestations and Symptoms

1. Red, itchy, and watery eyes.

2. Itchy nose. People who are allergic to pollen may also experience itchy eyes, ears and throat. Increased nasal discharge, mostly watery (sometimes dripping involuntarily). With inflammation, the nasal discharge thickens.

3. Blockage of the nasal canal. This happens intermittently or constantly, on one or both sides, with uneven degrees of severity.

4. Muffled hearing.

5. Sneezing. Bouts of sneezing happen more than three times daily, often in the morning or at night, or right after contact with the allergen.

6. Dark circles under the eyes.

7. A decreased sense, or even complete loss of smell.

Hand Reflexology and Acupressure

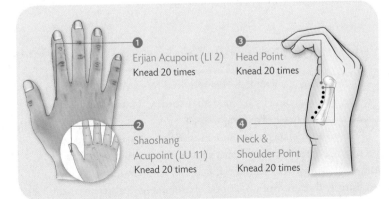

❶ Erjian Acupoint (LI 2)
Knead 20 times

❷ Shaoshang Acupoint (LU 11)
Knead 20 times

❸ Head Point
Knead 20 times

❹ Neck & Shoulder Point
Knead 20 times

Hand Exercises

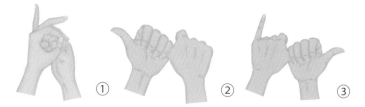

① ② ③

1. Bring the five digits of your right hand together and wrap them with the palm of your left hand. Squeeze and release them repeatedly.
2. Your left hand holds onto your right thumb, and pull it away slowly and with force.
3. The four fingers of the right hand hold onto the left thumb, and pull it away slowly and with force.

Other Methods

Patients with allergic rhinitis should pay attention to what they eat:

Avoid the following food: Unusually cold food, which will reduce your immune system and cause irritation in the respiratory tract; pungent and spicy food such as chili pepper and wasabi, which will irritate the respiratory mucosa; processed or refined food; artificial coloring, particularly Yellow No. 5.

Eat more: Food rich in Vitamins C and A, such as spinach, cabbage, bok choy, and radish; food containing hot energy, such as ginger, garlic, chives, cilantro, sticky rice, Chinese yam, dates, lotus seeds, coix seeds, brown sugar, and longan.

7. Glaucoma

Glaucoma is an eye problem characterized by elevated pressure in the eye, accompanied by a blood-shot cornea, dilated pupil, severely reduced vision, headaches, and nausea.

Congenital glaucoma occurs in those who have anatomical problems such as small eyeballs, short axial length, hyperopia, and shallow anterior chamber. If coupled with emotional swings, uncontrolled consumption of food, extreme physical strain, insufficient sleep, excessively long periods in dim light, and excessively long periods of reading with the head lowered down, glaucoma is likely to develop.

Secondary glaucoma is mostly caused by trauma, inflammation, hemorrhage, and tumors, which damage the angle of the eye chambers so that the drainage system does not function properly, resulting in increased pressure in the eye.

Manifestations and Symptoms

Acute angle-closure glaucoma: Blurred vision and the appearance of rainbow-colored circles around bright lights; pain in the eye and the head, nausea and vomiting, constipation, and rising blood pressure. Such systemic symptoms are easily confused with symptoms of other diseases such as gastritis, encephalitis, enteritis, and tension headaches. If left untreated, the patient may lose vision within 24 to 48 hours.

Chronic glaucoma: Slow progress, with eye pressure rising gradually. When the pressure is high, the patient may experience a slight headache, as well as soreness and swelling of the eyes. In addition to the shrinking of the optic nerve head, advanced glaucoma also manifests as a dilated pupil and cloudy cornea.

Hand Reflexology and Acupressure

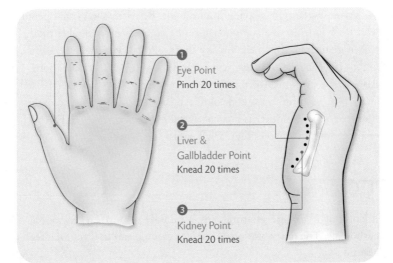

❶ Eye Point
Pinch 20 times

❷ Liver &
Gallbladder Point
Knead 20 times

❸ Kidney Point
Knead 20 times

Hand Exercises

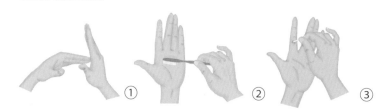

1. Align the four fingers side by side and hold them out against the center of the other palm (vertical). Swing left and right to jab the center of the palm.

2. Brush the center of the palm up and down with a toothbrush 30 times.

3. Spread out the five digits, and use a stick to jab the proximal and middle phalanges of the index finger in even dots.

Other Methods

People with glaucoma should maintain a healthy lifestyle.

First of all, make sure you sleep enough. Inadequate sleep and insomnia can result in rising eye pressure, inducing glaucoma. For the elderly, soak and wash your feet with warm water, and drink some milk before bed to ensure a good night's sleep. For people who are already experiencing eye pressure, ample sleep is necessary.

Avoid working or playing in dim light. Research shows that people who work in front of a computer for nine hours or more double their risk of glaucoma. If you are already short-sighted, you are at an even higher risk, and should have regular and thorough eye examinations. Also, if you work mostly in front the computer, clean your screen often, and adjust the brightness and color to a comfortable level. Also make sure that your computer is in a comfortable location. Most importantly of all, examine your eyes regularly for early detection of glaucoma.

8. Cataract

A clouding of the eye's natural lens, a cataract is caused by metabolic pathogens. The deterioration of the lens capsule can lead to impaired vision.

Manifestations and Symptoms

Congenital cataracts: Lens opacity at birth, often found in infants or young children. The cloudiness of the vitreous body is not total, and will not progress. The level of impact on the vision is determined by the location and the degree of the cloudiness.

Traumatic cataracts: This occurs after the lens capsular bag is either penetrated or burst. The former is penetration trauma, while the latter is blunt trauma.

Age-related cataracts: Often manifested as progressive blurred vision of both eyes among people who are 45 or older. During an eye examination, some grey cloudiness is detected in the pupil.

Hand Reflexology and Acupressure

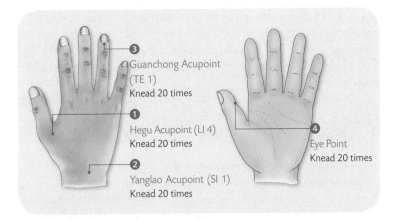

Guanchong Acupoint (TE 1)
Knead 20 times

Hegu Acupoint (LI 4)
Knead 20 times

Yanglao Acupoint (SI 1)
Knead 20 times

Eye Point
Knead 20 times

Hand Exercises

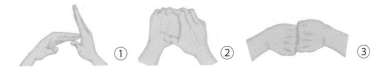

1. Align the four fingers side by side and hold them against the center of the other palm (vertical). Swing left and right to jab the center of the palm.

2. Form a tight fist with the left hand, and wrap the back of the fist with the right hand. Your right thumb presses and rubs the skin on

the back of the left hand.

3. With the palms facing down, form fists with both hands. Interlock the knuckles, and press them into the depressions of the other fist with force.

Other Methods

Avoid intense UV light. Wear sunglasses with UV protection if you need to go out.

Limit your calorie intake. Research has found that an obese person has a 30 percent greater chance of cataracts than a person of normal weight.

If you have had cataract surgery, do not lift heavy objects or do intense exercise within one or two months; avoid spicy and irritating food, and do not smoke or drink alcohol. Have weekly follow-up consultations after surgery, and wear protective eye masks. If your eyes are red and swollen, and if you feel pain in the eyes or experience declining vision, go back to the clinic immediately for consultation. Your vision will usually stabilize within two to four weeks after the surgery.

9. Acute Conjunctivitis

Acute conjunctivitis is an infection of the conjunctiva caused by repeated contact with air irritants and other allergens. It is most common in spring and summer, and symptoms will subside in late fall when the weather cools down. It is generally believed that the onset is related to such allergens as pollen, hair, sunlight, and dust. Although not contagious, it may trigger other allergies.

Manifestations and Symptoms

1. Redness of the conjunctiva: The closer to the corneal vault, the more evident the redness is. Blood vessels are winding and irregular, shaped like a net.

2. Sticky or pus-like discharge from the eyes, crusting over the eyelashes and making it hard to open the eyes first thing in the morning.

3. If the condition is mild, you will feel an itch or a burning sensation in one or both eyes, as well as a gritty feeling; if more severe,

you may be sensitive to light and experience runny eyes and heavy eyelids.

4. You may feel a swollen lymph node in front of your ear or under your jawbone.

Hand Reflexology and Acupressure

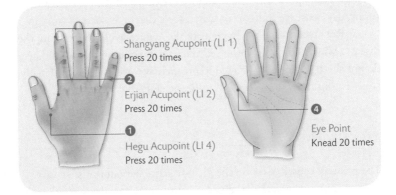

Shangyang Acupoint (LI 1)
Press 20 times

Erjian Acupoint (LI 2)
Press 20 times

Hegu Acupoint (LI 4)
Press 20 times

Eye Point
Knead 20 times

Hand Exercises

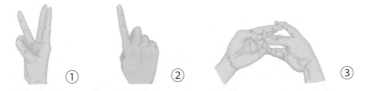

1. Form the finger-counting sign for "2," then abruptly stretch out the ring finger 10 times.

2. Stretch your hand flat with the palm facing away from you; quickly withdraw your thumb, middle finger, ring finger, and little finger, leaving only the index finger raised.

3. Press the left little finger with both thumbs while your left index finger moves toward the middle finger and touches it; your right index finger holds onto the left middle finger. Keep it this way for 18 minutes.

Other Methods
1. If you have acute conjunctivitis, wear goggles to avoid direct eye

contact with the water when swimming, as the pool water contains chlorine. The higher the chlorine content, the more irritating the water is to the eyes. Such irritation may lead to non-contagious conjunctivitis. If the water has a lower chlorine content, there is likely to be more bacteria, which may result in contagious conjunctivitis.

2. After swimming, wash your hands before taking off your goggles; then apply anti-inflammatory eye drops. If the eyes are red, runny, dry, sensitive to light, or gritty, see a doctor as soon as you can.

3. Pay attention to the hygiene of the eyes to avoid contracting the disease: Wash your hands often; if someone in your family has pinkeye, do not share potentially infected items such as towels and soap. Finally, stop visiting the swimming pool until the epidemic subsides.

10. Toothache

The primary causes of toothache include acute periodontitis, acute pulpitis, gum or periodontal abscess, acute gingivitis, dry socket syndrome, pain due to food lodged in the teeth, sensitive teeth, jaw tumors, and trigeminal neuralgia.

Manifestations and Symptoms

Toothache due to periapical periodontitis: Constant voluntary aching, radiating toward the head and the temple on the same side; the tooth feels as if it is growing longer; pain when chewing; evident pain when the teeth knock against each other lightly; swollen lymph nodes under the jaw; pain increases when pressed.

Toothache due to pulpitis: Spontaneous intermittent pain, which may radiate to the head and face on the same side, becoming severe during the night. It is hard to locate the affected tooth as the onset occurs; cold and hot stimuli may exacerbate the pain; light tapping of the tooth causes pain.

Toothache due to periodontitis: Red and swollen gum, oozing pus, bleeding; loose and weak teeth.

Toothache due to trigeminal neuralgia: Intermittent electrifying, stabbing, or prickling pain that lasts between ten seconds and one minute.

Hand Reflexology and Acupressure

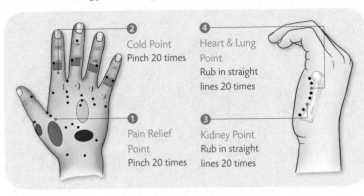

2 Cold Point
Pinch 20 times

4 Heart & Lung Point
Rub in straight lines 20 times

1 Pain Relief Point
Pinch 20 times

3 Kidney Point
Rub in straight lines 20 times

Hand Exercises

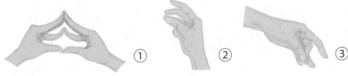

1. With five pairs of fingers facing each other, press the tips against each other to form the largest possible angle.

2. Bend the fingers of your right hand slightly, forming a hollow fist. Pinch the tips of your thumb and ring finger together.

3. Bend the five digits of your left hand slightly, forming a hollow fist. Pinch the tips of your thumb and the middle finger against each other.

Other Methods

Pay attention to oral hygiene in daily life, e.g., brush your teeth in the morning and at night, rinse your mouth after meals; avoid eating anything sweet before going to bed; avoid eating spicy and irritating food.

If you have no painkillers at hand, try the following methods to alleviate the pain:

1. Rub the Hegu acupoint (see page 20) with cold water or press it with your fingers.

2. If the tooth is sensitive to anything hot, there may be a buildup of pus in it. In this case, put a cold compress on the cheek and the pain will be alleviated.

Index